Sexually transmitted diseases

THE FACTS

BY

DAVID BARLOW
M.A.,B.M.,M.R.C.P.

Consultant Physician, Department of
Genito-urinary Medicine, St. Thomas Hospital, London

Cartoons by DICKINSON

Illustrations by TOM TREASURE M.S.,F.R.C.S.

OXFORD
OXFORD UNIVERSITY PRESS
NEW YORK · TORONTO

Oxford University Press, Walton Street, Oxford OX2 6DP

OXFORD LONDON GLASGOW
NEW YORK TORONTO MELBOURNE WELLINGTON
KUALA LUMPUR SINGAPORE JAKARTA HONG KONG TOKYO
DELHI BOMBAY CALCUTTA MADRAS KARACHI
NAIROBI DAR ES SALAAM CAPE TOWN

© David Barlow 1979

© Cartoons, Geoffrey Dickinson 1979

Reprinted 1981

British Library Cataloguing in Publication Data

Barlow, David
  Sexually transmitted diseases. – (Oxford medical
  publications).
  1. Venereal diseases
  I. Title   II. Series
  616.9'51   RC200   79-40381

  ISBN 0-19-261157-7

Set by Hope Services, Abingdon
and printed in Great Britain by
Richard Clay (The Chaucer Press), Ltd.,
Bungay, Suffolk

Contents

Acknowledgements

I would like to express my thanks to Dr W. Barlow, Dr J. Barrow, and Dr M.A.E. Symonds for advice and criticism of the manuscript; to Dr W.F. Felton, many of whose ideas I have borrowed when dealing with the epidemiology of gonorrhoea; and to the Photographic Department and the Departments of Microbiology and Virology at St Thomas's Hospital.

During the preparation of the manuscript, I have been much helped by reference to the *British Journal of Venereal Diseases*, the *Journal of the American Venereal Disease Association*, *Venereal diseases* by King and Nicol, Bailliere Tindall (1975) and *Recent advances in sexually transmitted diseases* by Morton and Harris, Churchill Livingstone (1975).

Introduction

This book is called *Sexually transmitted diseases: the facts* rather than *Venereal diseases: the facts*, because the venereal diseases are few in number. The reason for this is an accident of labelling rather than a reflection of incidence, because in most countries, including Great Britain, the venereal diseases are restricted to the two most well known, syphilis and gonorrhoea, with the occasional addition of lymphogranuloma venereum (LGV) or chancroid. In this country there is a further category of 'sexually transmitted diseases', which includes ten or so conditions that are acquired in the same way as the legally defined venereal diseases, the difference between 'VDs' and 'STDs' being a semantic rather than a practical or biological one.

In 1979 there will be over 1 million patient-visits to departments of genito-urinary medicine or venereology in England alone, representing a total of 350 000 separate diagnoses, by no means all of which, however, will be of a sexually transmitted infection. Great Britain and

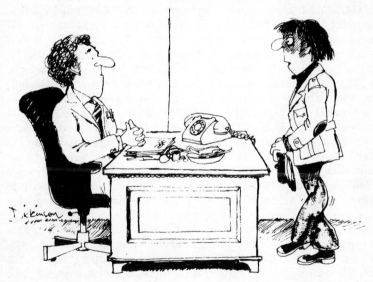

'It's not for me doctor — I'm inquiring for a friend.'

Ireland are the only countries in the world to have made a separate medical specialty out of the study, diagnosis, and treatment of the sexually transmitted diseases, and this is reflected in a lower incidence

1

of infection and a generally higher standard of patient care and clinic facilities than is found elsewhere.

If this book had been written thirty years ago, more space would need to have been devoted to the late effects of venereal disease. Nowadays, involvement of the cardiovascular and neurological systems by syphilis is rare, and congenital syphilis is likewise uncommon. Since the advent of antibiotics, the ravages associated with the late complications of syphilis and gonorrhoea no longer present a great problem, although the number of infections is not greatly different from that of the pre-antibiotic era. However, if the 'traditional' diseases have become more manageable, there has been no concomitant reduction in the problems posed by the sexually transmitted diseases. This is largely due to the recognition that many more infections can be considered as sexually transmitted than was the case even fifteen or twenty years ago.

The formal list of diseases which have to be notified to the Department of Health and Social Security each quarter by all the clinics in England comprises syphilis, gonorrhoea, chancroid, lymphogranuloma venereum, granuloma inguinale, non-specific genital infection, trichomoniasis, candidiasis, scabies, pubic lice, herpes genitalis, genital warts, and molluscum contagiosum. However, this list, while having the mark of Government approval and being longer than that of any other country, is probably not exhaustive enough. These days one would certainly add some viral infections, including hepatitis and cytomegalovirus, and several gut infections, to the list of diseases in which the sexual mode of transmission is an important one, particularly in male homosexuals.

The agents responsible for the sexually transmitted diseases include representatives of most types of micro-organism ranging in size from the smallest, the viruses, through the bacteria, to single-celled protozoa and even insects. The one factor that the majority of these diseases have in common is that only very rarely does protective immunity follow the first attack. This is in contrast to many other communicable diseases. It is unusual to suffer from measles, rubella, mumps, or yellow fever more than once. This is because the initial infection stimulates the body to produce effective antibodies, which not only eliminate the infection but also protect against reinfection at a later date. Not so the sexually transmitted diseases. You can be cured of gonorrhoea one morning with an appropriate antibiotic treatment and catch it again the same evening. This is true of all the other sexually transmitted infections, with the exception of herpes and viral hepatitis, which, while you may not *catch* them again, may be very difficult to eliminate from the body.

Whereas some organisms, such as those responsible for gonorrhoea and trichomoniasis, have adapted so much that they are transmitted only with difficulty by other than sexual means, others, like pubic lice and scabies, need only close contact, not necessarily of a sexual nature, to facilitate their transmission.

1

Sexual anatomy and function

In this chapter I shall describe the genital region in man and woman and discuss some aspects of normal sexual function and variations in sexual behaviour.

Anatomy

The first two illustrations show the normal appearances of the male and female external genitalia, the male being uncircumcised. There are, of course, considerable variations in the shape, size, and appearance of the genitalia and any such differences should not be regarded as abnormal.

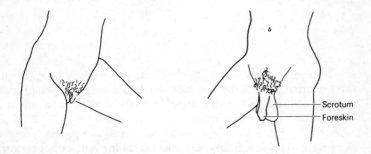

The male. The *penis* (from the Latin, tail) has both an excretory and a reproductive function. It is made up of three cylinders, two *corpora cavernosa* and one *corpus spongiosum*. These three cylinders are composed of erectile tissue, which, like the clitoris in the female, has the ability to shut off its drainage of blood and become swollen, hard, and erect. At the end of the corpus spongiosum (through which runs the urethra) is the *glans penis* which is larger than the rest of this cylinder and is the most sensitive part of the penis. It is normally covered by the foreskin, or *prepuce*, in the uncircumcised male. The skin covering the penis is loose in order to accommodate the considerable increase in

3

volume of the organ when erection occurs. There is surprisingly little variation in the size of the erect penis, although flaccid organs may differ considerably in appearance.

The *urethra* is the pipe through which the urine or ejaculate passes. It is about eight inches in length and runs from the urinary bladder, through the prostate gland, under the front of the pelvis, and, passing through the corpus spongiosum, it ends at the tip of the glans penis in an opening called the *urethral meatus*. There are many ducts and glands opening into the urethra, and it is the urethra which is the site of infection or inflammation in urethritis.

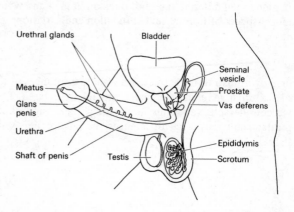

The *urinary bladder* in both sexes acts as a halfway house or store for the urine secreted by the kidneys. It is a muscular organ, which, when it contracts, forces the urine down the urethra. Infection inside the bladder is known as *cystitis*.

The *testis* (testicle, ball) serves as the factory for production of the male seed, the spermatazoa, and also makes the hormones responsible for the development of adult sexual characteristics, such as pubic hair, enlarged genitalia, beard, and deep voice. The testes are enclosed in the *scrotum*, a small muscular bag which hangs under the penis. Once they have been manufactured, the sperms are stored in the *epididymis*, which is a coiled tube attached to the side of the testis. The epididymis then joins with the *vas deferens* which winds a tortuous course in front of the pubic bone to join the urethra near its junction with the bladder. Just before it joins the urethra, the vas sprouts a small sac, the *seminal vesicle*, once thought to be a store for spermatazoa but now believed to be simply another gland which adds its secretion to the ejaculate. Male sterilization, vasectomy, involves cutting the vas deferens on each side, thereby preventing spermatazoa manufactured in the testes from reaching the urethra. The vas deferens is about 18 inches long, the same length as the thigh bone.

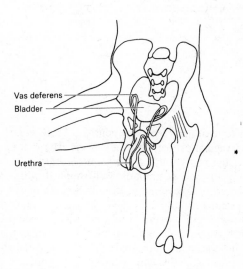

There are several glands associated with the urethra, which (like the seminal vesicles) produce secretions that, added to the spermatazoa, make up the ejaculate. The largest and most important of these is the *prostate gland*. The prostate encircles the urethra just after its emergence from the bladder and can be involved in infection, known as either acute or chronic prostatitis. It is the prostate gland which, when it enlarges in later life, as it often does, may cause difficulty in passing urine. Other smaller glands contribute mucous secretions to the ejaculate, and, like the prostate, may be involved in infection. Urethritis, from whatever cause, may be more difficult to clear up if these various glands are involved as well.

The female. Although it might seem highly unlikely, there are considerable similarities between the male and female genital anatomy — the different structures having started from similar beginnings during the development of the foetus of either sex. The differentiation of male or female characteristics is determined by the influence of sex hormones, which are present from a very early stage of development.

5

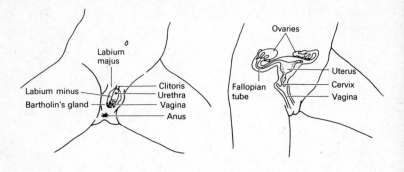

The female external genitalia consist of the *vulva*: the urethral opening, the vaginal orifice, and the *clitoris*. The clitoris is the female equivalent of the penis and it has a *glans clitoridis*, which corresponds to the glans penis and is similarly well supplied with sensory nerves. There are two corpora cavernosa clitoridis, and the organ, like the penis, erects under sexual stimulation. There is a small hood, corresponding to the foreskin, which lies over the clitoris. The female urethra is much shorter than that of the male. Its opening is just below the clitoris. This short length of the female urethra, combined with the closeness of the vagina and anus, explains why women are so much more prone to infections of the bladder than are men.

Below the urethral meatus is the orifice of the vagina, surrounded on each side by small folds of skin called the *labia minora*. The larger hair-covered lips outside the labia minora are called the *labia majora*. In the lower third of each labium minus is the small opening of *Bartholin's gland*, which produces a viscid secretion to aid lubrication in sexual intercourse. Infection involving these glands is called Bartholinitis and can be exquisitely painful. A few centimetres behind the vaginal opening lies the *anus*.

The *vagina* (in Latin, a sheath or scabbard) is about four inches long and lies between the urethra and bladder in front and the rectum behind. The upper third of the vagina is pierced by the neck of the womb, the *cervix uteri*, usually referred to simply as the cervix. This is the thin end of the inverted-pear-shaped *uterus* in which the fertilized egg (or *ovum*) develops. At its top the uterus is two inches across, and from each side come the *fallopian tubes*, themselves about 4½ inches in length, which serve as the channel down which the ovum travels from the *ovaries*, which are situated at the far end of the fallopian tubes. Infection of the tubes is called salpingitis. Such infection is one of the most important

6

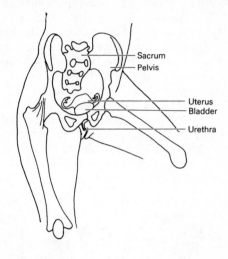

causes of infertility. The ovaries are the female equivalent of the male testes but are rather more economical in their production of seed, each releasing one egg every other month. Like the testes, the ovaries are responsible for producing sex hormones.

Function

The male. Erection of the penis occurs during conscious sexual stimulation, and also, involuntarily, during sleep. The nerves responsible for erection cause dilatation of the arteries supplying the erectile tissue in the penis and constriction of the veins which drain the organ, so that blood is trapped and the penis stiffens and becomes erect. These nerves, like the nerves responsible for ejaculation, are not under conscious control, being part of the so-called 'autonomic' nervous system. It is for this reason that man does not have as much control over erection or ejaculation as he might like. When ejaculation occurs the contents of the epididymis, the stored spermatazoa, are ejected along the vas deferens into the urethra where other muscles pump them out through the urethral meatus. At the same time the prostate gland, seminal vesicles, and other glands contribute their secretions to the ejaculate. Special muscles at the neck of the bladder contract to prevent flow back into the bladder. There are an estimated 300 million sperms in each ejaculate, of which, of course, only one will eventually fertilize the ovum of the female.

7

The female. Every month during the reproductive years, the uterus prepares to receive a fertilized ovum by building up a velvety, blood-rich lining. If implantation of a fertilized egg does not occur, this lining breaks down and is expelled from the uterus. This blood and tissue loss is called *menstruation* and the day that this menstrual flow starts is traditionally the first day of the menstrual cycle. Although menstrual cycles vary quite considerably in length from person to person, the average length is about 28 days with the 'period' taking up the first five or six of these. In such a 28-day cycle, *ovulation*, the release from the ovary of an egg into the fallopian tube, would occur on day 14, 14 days from the beginning of the next cycle. In a 35-day cycle, ovulation would occur on day 21, again 14 days from the start of the next cycle. It is for only about two days either side of the time of ovulation that fertilization and conception can take place.

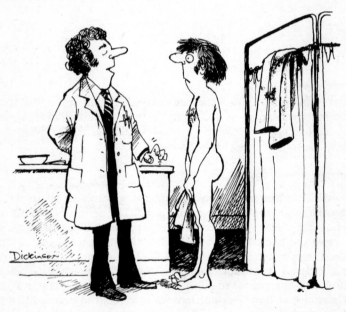

'I'm afraid I've got some bad news for your friend.'

The female adopts a more passive role in conception than the male, and physiologically she has less to do. Her reproductive role at this stage is simply to receive the male ejaculate containing the sperms, and to this end, during the period of sexual excitement before intercourse, various glands secrete mucus to aid lubrication and facilitate the insertion of the erect penis into the vagina.

8

Variations in sexual behaviour. This rather bald account has left out the intense excitement felt by both sexes, the progression to orgasm and the various positions and techniques that may be used. These are dealt with in a multitude of books on love-making. However, there are certain variations in sexual behaviour which have a direct bearing on sexually transmitted diseases and the likelihood of passing these on or acquiring them.

Oral sex, although mentioned in literature and depicted in art spanning millenia, has been thought of and described by many people as a perversion of sexual practice. Nowadays, the majority of people would regard it as a perfectly natural variation to be indulged in should both partners feel like it. *Fellatio* is the oral stimulation of the penis and *cunnilingus* is the oral stimulation of the clitoris and vulva by the sexual partner, male or female. Only in the last ten or so years has it been realized that infection can be spread quite easily by these practices and may pose problems as far as treatment is concerned. *Herpes simplex* virus infection (cold sores) can easily be transferred from the mouth to the genitalia, and since doctors have started looking for them, cases of gonococcal infection in the throat have been found in increasing numbers.

Male homosexuality is increasingly regarded as a variation of sexual behaviour rather than a perversion, and although the homosexual male is still treated badly by the law, in comparison to the heterosexual, he no longer feels the urgent need for anonymity and secrecy. The male homosexual is not immune to the sexually transmitted diseases; far from it, for the prevalence of these diseases is higher amongst homosexuals than in any other group, except possibly some groups of prostitutes. The reasons for this are not clear, but at the present time two diseases in particular, syphilis and type-B viral hepatitis, seem to be largely the preserve of the male homosexual. Rectal intercourse and fellatio are both common among homosexuals and diseases are therefore often to be found in the rectum and mouth. Anal or rectal intercourse is not, of course, confined to homosexuals — it is certainly practised by a sizeable minority of heterosexual couples as well. One recent survey in London showed that rectal intercourse, or attempts at it, had occurred in 35 per cent of sexually active women attending a clinic, during the preceding 6 months. It is probably an occasional rather than a regular feature of most people's sex lives. One rather strange anomaly is that such intercourse is legal between consenting male adults over the age of 21, but is illegal between heterosexuals and is punishable by a large fine or four years in prison. There seems to be virtually no problem of sexually transmitted infection among lesbians, unless one or other partner also indulges in heterosexual activity as well.

2

History and development
of a service

Historical aspects

There has always been considerable social stigma attached to the venereal diseases, probably more so in the country than the town. The following is an extract from the Manchester Quarter Sessions in 1651:

... to the Right worshipful Justices of the Peace and quorum for the County pallatyne of Lancaster
Right worshipfulls
This may be to acquaynt you that their is a pore yong women in oure Towne of Asston-underlyne infected with a filthy deceassed called the French poxe and shee saith shee was defiled by one Henry Heyworth a maryed man, but soe it is the report of that dessease occasioneth neighbours to deny hir harbour and shee is enforced to lye in the streetes and in great danger to bee starved, I do humbly intreate your worshipps to take it into your consideration and to grant your Order that the pore woman may be provyded for to prevent starveing, either upon the parrish charges, or upon the Costs of the said Heyworth whom she saith hath spoiled hir, whether yiur worshipps shall think fitt

The court was obviously not without compassion, for its judgement was: 'to erect some small cottage or Cabin for her in regard to her lothesomenes'.

Syphilis and its origin are subjects that have occupied physicians and historians over the ages perhaps more than any other condition. One of the major debates has hinged on the question of Columbus's, or rather his crew's, role in the pandemic of syphilis at the end of the fifteenth century. The so-called Columbian school maintain that syphilis was endemic to North America and that members of the crew of Columbus's first expedition acquired the infection and brought it back to Barcelona in 1493. A contemporary physician in Barcelona, Dr Diza de Isla, wrote that syphilis had been unknown until that date and that he had treated members of the crew for 'bubas' and the 'serpentine disease'. In 1494 Charles VIII of France crossed the Alps into Italy and undertook the siege of Naples. Some of the infected Spaniards joined his army as mercenaries and the massive spread of the disease throughout Europe stemmed from this time.

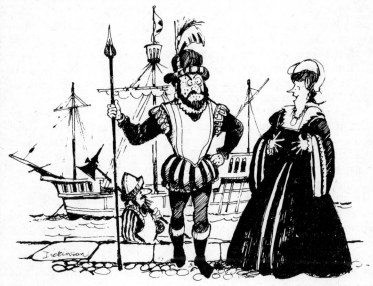

'What have you brought me back from the New World this time?'

In the spring of 1495 a dreadful plague broke out among those involved in the siege of Naples, bringing the siege to an end and resulting in disorganized retreat. The mercenaries from Spain and elsewhere made their way back home, spreading the disease as they went. The blame for syphilis was invariably ascribed to foreigners, with the result that the English called it the French disease, the French called it the Italian disease, the Italians, unable to make up their minds, called it both the French disease *and* the Spanish disease, while the Spanish called it the disease of Hispaniola (Haiti). Whoever's fault it actually was, the French aggressors, perhaps appropriately, were eventually blamed, for syphilis was generally referred to thereafter as the 'morbus gallicus'.

The pre-Columbian school cites evidence from ancient bones in Europe and North Africa to show that syphilis was extant long before Columbus's expeditions. It can also be argued that there are many references in the Old Testament to conditions that may well have been syphilis. In Deuteronomy, Moses threatened those who disobeyed the laws with the 'Botch of Egypt' which, apart from scabs and emerods, whatever they might have been, progressed to madness, blindness, and astonishment of heart. When it is said in Psalms that the enemies will be smitten in the 'hinder parts' it has been throught by many people to refer to haemorrhoids, but the description could equally refer to the anal manifestations of secondary syphilis, condylomata lata. Brim's translation 'You will be smitten with the Egyptian dermatitis, characterized by swellings, dry crusts, and ulcers, from which you will never be healed, and the Lord shall smite you in the knees, and in the legs, with a sore botch that cannot be healed from the sole of thy foot to the top of thy head' not only gives a description that would do very well for syphilis but also pre-empts the habit of the fifteenth-century Europeans of ascribing the disease to the enemy.

When the children of Israel were camped in Moab near Jericho, many of them came to worship the local god, Bael-Poor, and there was some mixing with the Moabites. As a result of this, a plague struck the Israelites which could have been venereal in origin. After the Moabite armies had been wiped out, all of the enemy women 'that have known man by lying with him' were ordered to be killed, a public health measure of a rather drastic order, although one that was highly effective.

There are several references to what may have been congenital syphilis. The visiting of the iniquity of their fathers on to succeeding generations in the Third Commandment, the banning of 'he that hath a flat nose', and the writing 'the fathers have eaten a sour grape and the children's teeth are set on edge' are suggestive of the stigmata of congenital syphilis.

Other theories on the origin or evolution of syphilis and the other diseases caused by similar organisms suggest that different populations have their own endemic treponemal disease, be it yaws, pinta, or syphilis, the presence of which makes it hard for one of the others to establish itself. Thus in yaws-endemic areas, where the disease is largely spread non-venereally in childhood, there is little opportunity for syphilis to spread, because of the degree of cross-immunity in the community. Holders of this theory would suggest that syphilis was already established in Europe in pre-Columbian days and it was the increase in knowledge and the travel resulting from the Renaissance that made it appear as if a new disease had been introduced.

Evolution of treatment

In 1363, Guy de Chauliac invented an ointment for the treatment of scabies which contained, amongst other things, gum-resin, yellow lead oxide, extract of wild delphinium, old pig's fat, and one-ninth part mercury. This unlikely concoction was one of the more important pharmacological advances in the history of medicine, albeit for the wrong reasons. For four hundred years after this formulation, mercury was the main drug of choice in the treatment of syphilis. Whatever its effect on scabies, the unction certainly had a healing, if not curative, effect on the morbus gallicus and was dispensed not only by the physicians of the time but also by 'butchers, sow-gelders, farriers, and itinerant mountebanks'. Guy de Chauliac had pointed out that his ointment was not without dangers if used in too great a quantity. It gave excessive salivation, pains in the belly, and caused the teeth to drop out. While physicians advised sparing use of the ointment, the quacks prescribed it liberally to great effect and had usually passed on to the next town before the inevitable relapses and the not infrequent deaths — results of over-treatment — had occurred. The problem with mercury was that the curative dose was much too close to the lethal dose, and it was easy to make the patient worse as a result of treatment.

For a brief time in the sixteenth century, mercury was supplanted by an extract of the bark of a West Indian tree, Guaiacum. In 1519 Von Hutten, a poet, published *De Morbi Gallici Curatione per Administrationem Ligni Guaiaci* in which he described the tortures of mercury treatment and the blessed relief of this new extract. Fracastorius, in whose poem Syphilis, the shepherd, was cured by guaiacum, endorsed the product and it was all the rage until Von Hutten died at the age of 35 of late syphilis in spite of his alleged cure. Although it was relatively ineffective, the fact that it was considerably safer than mercury meant that it remained in the pharmacopoeia of many countries until the twentieth century.

Two other drugs were introduced in the sixteenth century, 'China root', an extract of *Smilax sinensis*, which was brought over from Goa by the Portuguese, and sarsaparilla from *Sassafras officinale*, an American plant. Until just before the First World War, a strong decoction containing sarsaparilla, calomel, cinnabar, anise, fennel, senna, and liquorice was warmed up and taken in quart doses daily for ten days. In spite of these other nostra, mercury remained the mainstay of treatment, and in 1537 Barbarossa, a notorius Algerian pirate, on hearing that Francis I of France had acquired syphilis, sent the king a present of pills made up from mercury, rhubarb, amber, musk, and flour. After this royal endorsement pills were all the vogue and all the side-effects and problems of mercury overdosage became rife again. Many physicians from that time forward were of the opinion that nearly all the late complications of syphilis were, in fact, the result of mercury poisoning.

One of the reasons for the slow advance in understanding syphilis and gonorrhoea was the belief that the two conditions were simply different manifestations of the same disease. In syphilis the disease affected the outside of the genitalia with sores and ulcers, while in gonorrhoea the infection was on the inside. It was a not unreasonable assumption that a man who developed a discharge a few days after intercourse followed by a chancre some weeks later, without further exposure, was suffering from separate stages of the same infection. It was not until 1838 that there was general acceptance that the two diseases were distinct. As a result of this misunderstanding, for three hundred years sufferers from gonorrhoea were treated with mercury with all the risks that that entailed.

John Hunter, one of the most eminent surgeons of the eighteenth century, was responsible for lending weight to the belief that syphilis and gonorrhoea were the same disease, as a result of a fateful experiment. He himself was convinced that they were separate entities, and decided to prove this once and for all by inoculating himself with pus from a patient with a gonococcal discharge. With a tragic stroke of luck that set venereology back many decades, the patient from whom he collected the pus was also suffering from syphilis, and Hunter went on to develop both gonorrhoea *and* syphilis. In spite of mercury treatment, Hunter developed syphilitic involvement of the heart, which caused his early death.

In 1732 Thomas Dover published a treatise in which he advocated *metallic* mercury as a treatment for a variety of medical complaints *apart from syphilis* and pointed out that, taken in this form, it did not cause the side-effects of other mercury compounds. The metallic mercury was voided naturally, unchanged, in the faeces. This treatment very quickly caught on amongst those prescribing for syphilis, but with some embarrassing results for those who took the treatment. Apart from finding globules of mercury in people's shoes, a contemporary commentator, and opponent of this form of treatment, describes two men who used the same tavern regularly and both having supped from their little bottles of mercury would smoke a pipe and down some wine. After they had left the tavern, there were always some globules of mercury on the floor which the charitable thought had spilt from their bottles, but the waiters knew had come from the men themselves. He tells also of a lady at a dance whose partner thought she had dropped her pearls only to find, much to his consternation and her confusion, that they were the ubiquitous globules of mercury.

Potassium iodide was a favoured treatment for syphilis for some time following the publication in the *Lancet* of a series of papers advocating its use. This new treatment did not have the unpleasant and dangerous side-effects of mercurial treatment and was hailed at the time, like many other 'new' treatments, as the long-awaited answer to the problems of syphilis. Arsenic compounds were introduced towards the end of the nineteenth century, but it was the introduction of arsphenamine, or salvarsan, in the early twentieth century that produced the first really viable alternative to mercury.

Shortly after that, malarial treatment of late neurological syphilis was brought in. For many years it had been thought that high fever had certain curative properties, and some patients were deliberately exposed to mosquitoes which were known to be carrying the malarial

14

parasite in the hope that the resulting infection and high temperature would have a beneficial effect on the disease process. Although this treatment was undoubtedly efficacious in some cases, the patients ended up with malaria, and so a 'fever box' was developed in which the patient's temperature could be maintained at over 106 °F for several hours. This treatment was not without risks, however, and careful temperature monitoring was vital, as a small rise above that recommended could result in the death of the patient.

Bismuth was introduced in the 1920s and finally ousted mercury from the therapeutic armamentarium, because its curative action could be attained with doses which, unlike those of mercury, did not approach the lethal amount. Bismuth is still used by some practitioners as an adjunct to penicillin therapy, but in most centres the advent of penicillin and other antibiotics has, at long last, brought an end to the many centuries during which the treatment of syphilis was worse than the disease itself.

Development of a service

Whatever else may be said about Britain's standing abroad, one indisputable fact, albeit a somewhat dubious distinction, is that, in the field of sexually transmitted diseases, this country leads the world. Which is not to say that such diseases are more common in this country or that the cases are more florid or medically interesting, simply that, for historical reasons, the delivery of both diagnosis and treatment is better than elsewhere.

Pre-dating the National Health Service by over thirty years, in 1916 the Venereal Disease Regulations were passed instructing all local health authorities to provide clinics for the diagnosis and treatment of the venereal diseases. These clinics were to be associated with local hospitals, and confidentiality and freedom from charge were mandatory. At the same time it was made illegal for anyone who was not fully medically qualified and registered to treat these diseases. This stipulation, supported by an Act of Parliament, is still in force, and, as far as treatment is concerned, puts the sexually transmitted diseases in a unique position. For, surprisingly, it is not illegal for other conditions to be treated by medically unqualified people as long as such people do not *claim* to be doctors. There is no legal reason why your next-door neighbour shouldn't take out your appendix, or you his, should either of you feel so inclined, though the premiums for third-party insurance might be prohibitively high.

Following the National Health Service Act of 1946, all the clinics were brought under the control of the Regional Hospital Boards and the Boards of Governors of the Teaching Hospitals. Thus, for over sixty years, there have been specially equipped and staffed clinics throughout the country, where patients can be seen without direct referral by their general practitioners. When prescription charges were introduced, the special clinics were exempted, and treatment continues to be free.

The other single most important factor responsible for raising the standard of care was the recognition of *venereology* as a clinical specialty in its own right. This meant that the clinics were run, in the main, by *trained* medical officers whose special interest and expertise could be concentrated on the sexually transmitted diseases. Apart from Southern Ireland, there is no country in the world that has an equivalent specialty, and, as a result, standards of diagnosis, treatment, and care abroad vary from the inadequate to the unbelievably bad in most cases.

The scope of the specialty of venereology has widened over the years, and following recommendations from the Royal College of Physicians has now been renamed 'genito-urinary medicine' to take into account the small proportion of patients attending the clinics who have a 'venereal disease'. It is felt that fewer people would be put off attending with other genital or sexual problems if the stigma of going to a 'VD' clinic could be dispensed with. Rather sadly, the sites allotted to these clinics were often away from the main hospital departments and were either to be found in dungeon-like basements or else in prefabricated huts. In the last ten or fifteen years there has been a trend away from this geographical separation of the clinic, and there are now several purpose-built departments above ground designed as integral parts of new hospital complexes.

Apart from a specialist service second to none, the importance of accurate figures relating to the incidence of the various conditions has not been overlooked, and, again, Great Britain leads the world. Perhaps because of the long-standing provision of special clinics, the large majority of cases of sexually transmitted disease are seen in such clinics, in contrast to other countries, where less than 20 per cent of cases are seen in hospitals. This has meant that elsewhere it has been very difficult to assess the extent of the problem, which has therefore been underestimated. Every clinic in the United Kingdom has to collect figures on the total attendance and the diagnoses and submit them quarterly to the Department of Health. With syphilis and gonorrhoea, the ages are also recorded, and this means that an accurate map of disease prevalence can be drawn and any trends or changes can be recognized very quickly.

It is accepted that some 10 to 15 per cent of cases are seen outside the clinics by private or general practitioners, and it is unusual for these cases to be reported to the Department of Health.

The development of the service for the diagnosis and treatment of the sexually transmitted diseases in Great Britain stems largely from the efforts of one man, Colonel L. W. Harrison, who, somewhat unwillingly, was posted to a Guards Regiment Hospital in Rochester Row, London, in 1909 as pathologist. This hospital had been converted to a centre for research and instruction in the venereal diseases, and, by a happy co-incidence, this was a time of great advances in the field. It had become possible to demonstrate the causative organism of syphilis, *Treponema pallidum*, under the microscope; there was soon to be available a blood test, the Wasserman Reaction (WR), which enabled syphilis to be diagnosed in the absence of any signs of the disease; and finally, a new syphilitic treatment, Salvarsan, an arsenic compound, had become available.

Until this time, the mainstay of treatment for syphilis had been mercury in some form or other, either by internal administration or in the form of unctions. The Special Advisory Board for the Army Medical Service had laid down as a basis for treatment 'a more or less continuous course of mercury by mouth for 1½ to 2 years' combined with mercurial ointment rubbed into the skin for 20 to 30 minutes daily over a six-week period. Other regimens involved treatment with iodine compounds.

Although Salvarsan was a considerable advance on previous treatments, it was not itself without risks and side-effects, and it was considered important to ensure that the 'C/T' ratio was 'propitious'. This ratio was derived by dividing the 'dose sufficient to destroy all parasites' by the 'maximum dose which will not kill the patient'! Notwithstanding the risks associated with this treatment, the discovery of Salvarsan was greeted throughout the world with great enthusiasm. One Russian paper, described as 'highly conservative', contained a piece, some of which, it was said at the time, was barely capable of being rendered into printable English. Having exalted over the 'liberation of whoredom' it went on to say, 'No more danger! Down with the family! No need to toil in the sweat of one's brow to support it! Long live prostitution – the like of which has not been seen since the downfall of Rome . . .'

Harrison and his team at Rochester Row did much of the pioneer work on Salvarsan and their discoveries were used with great benefit during the First World War. It was not just in the treatment of syphilis that advances were being made at this time. The current treatment of gonorrhoea was the use of strong antiseptic solutions, which were run into the urethra under considerable pressure with the idea of irrigating the urethra and washing out any pathogenic organisms. Harrison felt that the solutions used were too strong and suggested that the containers of irrigating fluid should be no more than three feet above the patient's pelvis, in contrast to the ten feet that had been the norm. Following this reduction in the head of pressure, the incidence of post-irrigation epididymitis was greatly reduced.

Sexually Transmitted Diseases

When war broke out in 1914, Harrison was sent to France to join the British Expeditionary Force and regarded this as a heaven-sent opportunity to move away from the subject of the venereal diseases. There had been no provision by the War Office for dealing with the problem of sexually transmitted diseases, the only directive having been an exhortation from Lord Kitchener to the troops to be sexually continent. The situation rapidly became chaotic, and a 250-bedded hospital, which had been allotted for these cases, contained some 1000 patients, when in 1915 Harrison was urgently called upon to sort things out.

Under Colonel Harrison's supervision, treatment regimens were brought under control, and by the spring of 1916 the hospital in Le Havre had 3000 beds. Shortly afterwards, Harrison was recalled to Rochester Row and was appointed Adviser in VD to the War Office.

As Adviser to the Ministry, Harrison was invited to take charge of a 'model' clinic at St. Thomas Hospital in London. This clinic embodied his four major principles which were:

(i) waiting periods should be kept to a minimum;
(ii) examination should be conducted in the greatest possible privacy and never in the presence of other patients;
(iii) there should be ease of access of staff to patients; and
(iv) the distances covered by staff and the time occupied in obtaining necessary instruments and drugs should be kept to a minimum.

This appointment as adviser of a practising physician in charge of a big, busy clinic was perhaps one of the major factors in the evolution of a co-ordinated service throughout the country. Harrison spent much time visiting other clinics up and down the country advising on how they might be run more efficiently. In addition to his clinical work, research, and advisory duties, Harrison was a founder member of the Medical Society for the Study of the Venereal Diseases and was joint editor of the *British Journal of Venereal Diseases* between 1925 and 1942.

He was instrumental in starting the Venereal Disease Reference Laboratory in 1924. The need for a centralized reference laboratory stemmed from the difficulty in persuading venereal-disease pathologists that their own test methods might need revising. Once it had been opened, it became possible to test patients' sera in parallel, thereby convincing other doctors that their tests could be improved.

3

Sexually transmitted diseases
world-wide

It is very difficult to compare statistical data from different countries, because of the variation in the criteria used for diagnosis and notification, and the greater or lesser degree of under-reporting that is found almost everywhere. The figures from the United Kingdom, acknowledged as they are to be the most accurate, still underestimate the true incidence of infection. What can be gathered from such figures as are available, are trends in disease prevalence and changes in the geographical patterns of infection.

There is a general feeling that syphilis, until recently thought to be almost under control, is now recrudescing. Apart from the People's Republic of China, which claims to have eradicated syphilis in the space of about ten years, most countries are now reporting an increase in the number of cases of early infectious syphilis, usually amongst male homosexuals. In areas where other treponematoses used to be endemic, as was yaws in the West Indies, the eradication of the non-venereal treponemal disease has been followed by an upsurge in the incidence of syphilis, perhaps because there is an ecological niche to be filled. Congenital and late syphilis, both neurological and cardiovascular, seem to be less common than in previous times.

If there is any doubt in the case of syphilis, there is none at all with regard to gonorrhoea. All five continents are involved in an increase in the incidence of gonorrhoea, which, in many cases, is now more common than during the pre-war period. In many countries gonorrhoea is the most commonly notified communicable disease, even allowing for the under-reporting, which usually far exceeds the notification rate. Added to this, there are several areas where the level of resistance to antibiotics among the gonococci makes it extremely difficult to treat.

Chancroid is generally less common than it used to be, and is very rarely seen in Northern Europe, although it still poses problems in Asia and parts of Africa. Lymphogranuloma venereum, once not uncommon in parts of Europe, notably Finland, Romania, and Spain, is now rarely seen except when imported from West Africa, the Caribbean, or South

America. Granuloma inguinale is evenly distributed in tropical regions, with a high prevalence in Papua New Guinea and Southern India and a few cases in Africa, the Southern USA, South-East Asia, and the Caribbean.

In most countries the other sexually transmitted diseases are not reported, but, where they are, there is said to be a general increase in all infections, particularly non-specific urethritis.

World-wide co-operation in the matter of the venereal diseases was first formalized by the Brussels agreement of 1924 when the signatories undertook to provide a free treatment service for seamen of all countries who were found to be suffering from infection. The World Health Organization took over the administration of this agreement in 1947, and has continued, since then, to advise on suitable antibiotics for treatment, and methods to be used in the blood tests for syphilis. They have also been responsible for many symposia and meetings for specialists in the field of venereology. In spite of these efforts, the incidence of the sexually transmitted diseases continues to increase. The trouble is that when two people hop into bed together, whether it is after a disco in the West End of London, in an igloo in Greenland, or in a hut in Africa, the last thing on their minds is the opinion of a collection of 'VD' experts from the WHO in Geneva.

While it is unquestionably a step in the right direction for such international teams to make recommendations as to optimal treatment schedules and ideal diagnostic facilities, it avails little if governments do not take their advice or if there is a shortage of money, personnel, or both. This appears, sadly, to be the situation in many countries, and suggestions like the one from the WHO document *Social and health aspects of sexually transmitted disease* (1977) that 'it is essential for clinics to have the basic equipment required for making rapid diagnosis: the darkfield examination, a quick micro-flocculation test for syphilis, and smear and culture of specimens for gonorrhoea' are not much use to a health worker in a village in India, who, far from considering buying a microscope, cannot obtain the antibiotics needed to cure gonorrhoea had he the facilities for diagnosing it. However, even if governments were prepared to spend more of their gross national product on health-care facilities, while the incidence of complications from the sexually transmitted diseases might decline, no amount of money would have a significant effect on the prevalence of these diseases unless it could be used to alter people's attitudes and behaviour.

Information about the success or otherwise of control measures in the Eastern bloc is scarce. There is evidence of good microbiological research emanating from Russia and Poland, but even if the communist countries had accurate figures on disease prevalence they might feel that publication of these would reflect badly on their political systems.

The alternative to keeping quiet about these problems is, of course, to deny their very existence, and the prize for the most successful campaign of VD eradication, or alternatively the rarest piece of dissembling, must go to Communist China which claims to have got rid of syphilis in the ten years after 1950.

According to one Chinese doctor writing in the *Journal of the American Venereal Disease Association* in 1975, the incidence of venereal disease was 4 per cent for town dwellers and 1 per cent for the rural population after the last war. As a result of a nation-wide campaign, they reduced the incidence of syphilis to one case in every ten million population in the mid-fifties and one case in every hundred million by 1960. The elimination of prostitution was a simple matter, the social revolution took care of that, but there remained the problem of infection in the population at large. They used two methods for this. First a questionnaire was distributed to all adults in China, and all those who had suspicious symptoms were subjected to the second procedure, which was a new simple blood-test that could be performed on farms or in factories, and gave an answer in twenty minutes. I quote:

Sexual liberation can only help spread VD. Among the Chinese people, Victorian morality ranks high in the world. Sex is not very important in the Chinese way of life. Extramarital relations are prohibited, both morally and legally. Illegitimacy also is illegal, for which both parties may be imprisoned . . . thus, a fundamental change in the social system, an effective system of mass public education, and a thorough disease control programme worked wonders in eliminating VD. Other countries have attempted to duplicate this success but so far, have failed.

If only it were so simple.

Both Africa and the Indian sub-continent suffer from the combined problems of over-population and a paucity of funds and personnel for health care. Although there are centres of excellence to be found, their contribution to reducing endemic levels of sexually transmitted diseases can be only minute when compared with the extent of the problem. It is in Africa and India that one can still find patients ravaged by the late complications of syphilis, gonorrhoea, and lymphogranuloma venereum, and any hopes of eventually controlling levels of infection will almost certainly depend on paramedical or 'barefoot' doctors' playing a larger role. What is worrying is that these countries may serve as reservoirs of infection should any of the richer countries ever get on top of their own VD problem. Already one is seeing cases with β-lactamase-producing gonococci in London which have been acquired in Ghana, and there is little hope of preventing their eventual spread throughout the community if no action is being taken in the source country.

An example of the futility of pouring money uncontrolledly into a

21

service is given by the United States, which has one of the highest rates of infection with the sexually transmitted diseases, one of the highest rates of resistance among its gonococci, and one of the highest, if not *the* highest, budgets for research and education into these diseases in the world. It is undeniable that a great deal of important and fundamental research has come from the several centres of excellence in the USA. The Centre for Disease Control in Atlanta, Georgia, is probably pre-eminent in terms of pure research into the organisms responsible for the sexually transmitted diseases, and yet none of this concentrated effort has had any effect on the levels of gonorrhoea or syphilis in America.

In 1971 following recommendations from both the World Health Organization and the International Union against the Venereal Diseases and Treponematoses (IUVDT), a travelling seminar of experts from all over the world was convened to examine the service for sexually transmitted diseases in the United States, the training of the medical personnel and undergraduates, and to suggest ways in which these could be improved. The impetus for this study came from the disastrous upsurge in the levels of these diseases, particularly gonorrhoea, which was increasing at 10 to 15 per cent. Among several comments and recommendations that this body made were:

— gonorrhoea was now the commonest communicable disease in the United States after the common cold, and its incidence was rising;
— it was quickly apparent that undergraduate medical education about the sexually transmitted diseases was inadequate and frequently non-existent, not being part of the standard medical-school curriculum;
— because the clinics were not attached to university medical schools, it was improbable that good physicians would be attracted to the specialty;
— not only was the undergraduate teaching poor, but there was only a minimal amount of postgraduate education in this subject; part of the reason for this was that there was a shortage of suitable qualified and experienced doctors who knew enough to take on such post-graduate teaching; and
— because the clinics were not attached to the main hospitals, there was no feedback from other disciplines in medicine, and, furthermore, the doctors working in the clinics did not have to undergo the vigorous selection procedures that were usual for hospital posts.

And so the list went on. It was a damning report on America's VD service by her international peers and colleagues, many of whom, it might be added, had little better to offer back in their own countries. However, the body of the report was accepted by the Americans, who if they needed any further confirmation were given it in the form of a 72 per cent failure rate among recently qualified army medical officers who had been given a questionnaire on the venereal diseases and their control. It seems that the situation in the United States today has changed little since 1971, apart from an increased awareness among the teachers in the medical schools that the long neglected subject of the sexually transmitted diseases should form a more important part of the medical curriculum.

If the situation in the United States is less than perfect, then the state of affairs on the other side of the Panama Canal could only be described as disastrous. Sexually transmitted diseases are very much more common among younger age groups, and in South America 50 per cent of the population is under 20. In Brazil this figure reaches 70 per cent. Self-medication without diagnosis is common, because antibiotics are freely available without prescription, and the reported figures for incidence of disease are thought to represent 1 per cent of the true case numbers. It has been estimated that there are 24 000 cases of gonorrhoea *each day* in South America, that is just under half the total yearly figures for England. It is not surprising that gonococcal eye infection in newborn babies, a good measure of undiagnosed infection in a community, is extremely prevalent. To quote one Brazilian professor, '*Everyone* over the age of three years has got scabies'. They do, however, run a yearly course in sexually transmitted diseases in Santiago, but it may well take more than that to make any impression at all on disease levels.

As is the case in the majority of countries in the world, none of the countries in the Common Market (with the exception of Southern Ireland) recognizes venereology or genito-urinary medicine as a distinct specialty. Most of the specialists are *Dermato*-venereologists, and usually only about 10 per cent of the patients they see are suffering from a sexually transmitted disease, the remainder having skin problems. Throughout the EEC it is the rule for patients with sexually transmitted diseases to attend a private doctor for their diagnosis and treatment, and these private practitioners do not report the cases that they have seen. As a result, the published national figures are generally gross underestimates.

France. As well as the large centres in places such as Paris and Lyons, there are clinics attached to universities, and in non-university towns there are local *dispensaires* at which the treatment is free. Although the treatment is free, the patient may well be asked to pay for the tests used in diagnosis, and for a woman who wished to be screened for, say, gonorrhoea, trichomoniasis, and candidiasis, the bill might come to 250 francs, without the blood tests for syphilis, and if she was unfortunate enough to have an ulcer that might be syphilitic or herpetic, a further 150 francs could be added to the bill. Once the diagnosis had

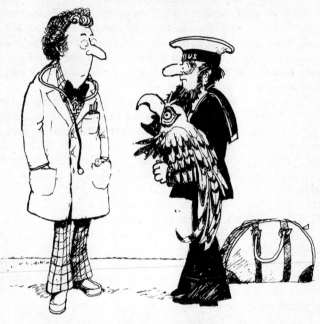

'I warned him about having a girl in every port.'

been made, only treatment for the recognized venereal diseases would be free, i.e. gonorrhoea, syphilis, chancroid, and LGV.

It is estimated that only 20 per cent of cases of sexually transmitted disease are seen in the specialist clinics. The curriculum at the medical schools does not make the study of dermato-venereology compulsory, and it is not unusual for a doctor to qualify in France having had little or no training in these subjects.

As regards the treatment and follow-up of cases of syphilis, the French, like the Italians, mostly subscribe to a 'continental' approach. Many years ago, when there were only relatively inaccurate and non-specific blood-tests for the diagnosis of syphilis, it was the aim of treatment to render these blood-tests negative and treatment would be continued with this end in view. With the evolution of more specific and sensitive tests, this ideal has become impossible. The newer blood tests may well remain positive indefinitely, following infection, and no amount of treatment will alter them. Blood-tests are now available to tell whether someone has had German measles in the past, and nobody in their right mind would suggest that such a positive blood test indicated the presence of *active* German measles long after the patient had recovered from the infection. However, the blood-tests for syphilis are

24

regarded in a different light, and prolonged courses of treatment may be prescribed, sometimes spanning several years, in a vain attempt to clear the blood of evidence of past syphilitic infection. The patients, with the spectre of inadequately treated syphilis hanging over them, naturally enough submit willingly to these lengthy, and expensive courses of treatment.

Denmark. The Danish system for dealing with sexually transmitted diseases is one of the better ones in Europe, and the impetus for this is provided by the State Serum Institute in Copenhagen. This large pathology institute regularly sends out to all doctors in Denmark special packs containing a transport medium into which samples from patients suspected of having gonorrhoea can be inoculated. They also enclose stamped addressed envelopes so that these samples can be returned to the Institute with little trouble. From this has developed an extremely high quality culture service, without which, as will be seen in the chapter on gonorrhoea, it is difficult to cope adequately with the disease, particularly in women. The Institute also deals with all the serological tests for syphilis for the whole of Denmark and they have a 'Wasserman' file, reminiscent of *1984*, in which the results of all such tests performed since 1920 are kept.

The Scandinavians in general have a much more open view of sex and the problems associated with it and have a less punitive approach than is seen in other countries. In the early seventies, the Swedes, worried by the startling increase in the number of cases of gonorrhoea, launched a health education campaign featuring a 'flying condom' which could be seen on all the best hoardings, exhorting the general public to use a protective in all acts of sexual intercourse. While this campaign was in force, Sweden was the only country to register a fall in the reported number of cases of gonorrhoea. The Danes have also taken a more enlightened viewpoint and have enlisted the help of a 'swinging' young poet to publicize their attempts at health education. They also introduced stickers to be attached to envelopes featuring a naked lady sitting cross-legged in a bed of flowers, a small heart covering her genitalia, with the inscription 'Love, not disease.'

There is compulsory sex education in schools and this must include at least half an hour on the sexually transmitted diseases. However, although the age of consent is fifteen, it is illegal to prescribe the oral contraceptive for someone of this age.

The treatments for gonorrhoea and syphilis are standardized throughout the country, and an estimated 80 per cent of cases are seen in the special dermato-venereological clinics. Their figures for the incidence of the various diseases are fairly accurate, every doctor having to fill in a form listing the number of cases of communicable disease seen each week; however, as elsewhere, the minor sexually transmitted diseases are not included. There are main clinics attached to all the university hospitals, and the training, both undergraduate and postgraduate, is thorough and comprehensive. Although the patient is expected to pay for his treatment, he will be reimbursed via the State medical insurance scheme.

Holland. Like Denmark, Holland is one of the more go-ahead countries with regard to the sexually transmitted diseases, but, lacking the centralized pathology laboratory, the standard outside the four clinics (two in Rotterdam and one each in Amsterdam and Utrecht — there are no provincial or peripheral clinics) is variable, with a few private practitioners providing the only reasonable alternative. Even in the university centres, perhaps only 50 per cent of cases are notified, while reporting from private practitioners is non-existent. The Dutch are unique in including non-specific urethritis on their contact slips along with the venereal diseases.

An interesting insight into the relative financial demerits of practising medicine in the United Kingdom is given by the difficulty the University at Rotterdam had in 1976 in filling an assistant professor's post in the venereal diseases, since the salary was *only* £22 000 and, working for an academic department, the scope for private practice was limited.

West Germany. The officially notifiable diseases are gonorrhoea, syphilis, LGV, and chancroid, but neither the hospital specialist nor the private practitioner reports the cases that he sees. The specialist in Germany is a dermato-venereo-andrologist, andrology being the male equivalent of gynaecology and including the diagnosis and treatment of male infertility and other genital disorders. There are 25 university and 25 municipal clinics, and the training of their specialists is both long and thorough. There are also a few special sailors' clinics in ports, but even so two-thirds of patients will be seen and treated by private practitioners.

Although the standard of service offered by the special clinics is generally fairly high, in some ways the Germans are still in the Dark Ages with regard to the sexually transmitted diseases. For instance, the distinction between gonorrhoea and non-specific urethritis is a blurred one, with much chronic urethritis being attributed to infection with 'pseudo-gonococci'. Since there are perfectly reliable and accepted micro-biological methods for distinguishing between *Neisseria gonorrhoeae* and the other members of the Neisserian family (apart from *N. meningitidis*, many other non-pathogenic members can be found on and in the human body), there is no justification for this bacteriological obfuscation.

Only the professor in a hospital department is allowed to do private practice and this must be done on the hospital premises. Although this exclusion of the junior consultant grades from private practice might well be unacceptable in this country, the Germans have recognized the usefulness of having the specialist readily available on the hospital site.

Italy. Italy shares with France a decidedly odd method, by English standards, of training medical students. Following the student riots in Paris in the late sixties, a certain anarchy crept into the medical course. This means that not all the subjects are compulsory, and, as in France, it is possible to qualify without having received any instruction in either dermatology or venereology.

There is a network of clinics throughout Italy — all towns with more than 50 000 inhabitants having one. However, the standard of the specialists is not necessarily very high and, as ever, many patients are seen privately, with a resulting underestimate of the true incidence of the various diseases. For example, in the last six months of 1975, only three cases of female gonorrhoea were reported from the province of Tuscany, which includes Florence with its large tourist trade and a local population of some two million. Since it is virtually impossible to obtain cultures for the gonococcus, the chances of making the correct diagnosis are considerably reduced. Only 2720 cases of gonorrhoea in both sexes were reported in 1972.

There is an odd ambivalence directed to matters sexual in what is recognized as a staunchly Roman Catholic country. The issue of whether to legalize abortion has brought down an Italian government, and yet the age of consent is fourteen, and furthermore sexual intercourse below that age is only illegal if the minor concerned brings charges. There is no law in Italy against doctors sleeping with their patients. Professor Giovanni Caletti, a dermato-venereologist who runs a centre for sex education near Venice, strongly believes that the way to combat the rising incidence of sexually transmitted diseases is by improved education rather than by improving the medical service available to an at-risk population. He produced in 1975 the results of a large survey, hailed as the 'Italian Kinsey report', in which he found that 50 per cent of Italian women and 25 per cent of men engaged in sex 'only to please' their partners; that 46 per cent of women and 19 per cent of men faked orgasm; and that 49 per cent of women and a surprising 32 per cent of men reported that they were virgins at marriage. In spite of this, 79 per cent of Italian men believed their wives to have been virgins when they married. Caletti's admirable attempt at removing fear, ignorance, and stigma from sexual topics is tempered slightly by his view that prostitution is 'disgusting' and that masturbation is not harmful as long as it is not indulged in *more than twice a month* (my italics).

Italy is not alone in believing that, because their reported figures for sexually transmitted diseases are low, they do not have a problem.

27

However, unless the undergraduate and postgraduate training are improved and more time, money, and thought are spent on the service, it is unlikely to improve. The standard textbook on the venereal diseases deals only with syphilis, gonorrhoea, chancroid, and LGV, with an addendum on NSU, and confuses the complications of non-specific urethritis with those of gonorrhoea.

Belgium. The notifiable venereal diseases in Belgium are syphilis, gonorrhoea, chancroid, and LGV, but there is a considerable degree of under-reporting, as witnessed by the official figures for 1975, which gave a total of 771 cases of gonorrhoea for the whole of Belgium. This figure is less than half the number of cases reported by *one* clinic, out of thirty odd, in London for that year. One of the main problems is that there is a clear separation between the various specialties, each of which has its own payment for a case. Thus a paediatrician is paid almost twice as much as a general practitioner for each patient that he sees, but less than a general physician, who is given twice as much as a dermato-venereologist. A psychiatrist is paid more than any other specialist. With this strict demarcation, syphilis will be treated by the dermato-venereologist, gonorrhoea by the urologist, and all female infections by the gynaecologist. Since the latter two specialists do not receive any special training in the sexually transmitted diseases, and neither will notify the cases that they see even if they manage to diagnose them, it is not surprising that chaos ensues.

There are clinics attached to all the university and large municipal hospitals, but the government has shut down the local clinics because they deny that there is any problem. This means that, effectively, there are clinics only in the larger cities. There is a body, the National League against the Venereal Diseases, which receives a grant from the government and organizes lectures in schools, prisons, and to the army, but it is clear that their efforts have little effect on the prevalence of disease. For many years the Government offered an annual award of 10 000 Belgian francs for research into sexually transmitted diseases, but even this has been discontinued, perhaps because the award always went to a foreigner.

Luxembourg. Although they recognize the specialty of dermato-venereology in Luxembourg, there is not one single clinic in the Grand Duchy. Since they do not have any medical schools, all medical students have to train outside Luxembourg in one of the countries whose medical degrees it recognizes. These are Switzerland, Germany, Belgium, and Austria.

There is a strong feeling against opening a special clinic in the city of Luxembourg itself, because of fears that it would be difficult to preserve anonymity. There is no contact-tracing as such, but, because it is felt that most of the problem is due to prostitutes (an unlikely truth

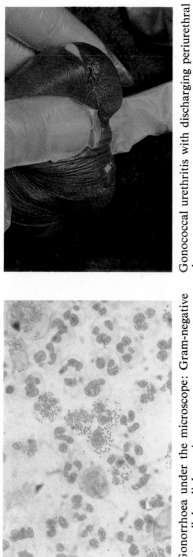

Gonococcal urethritis with discharging periurethral abscess

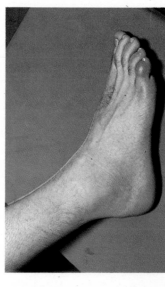

Involvement of ankle joint in gonococcal septicaemia

Gonorrhoea under the microscope: Gram-negative intracellular diplococci

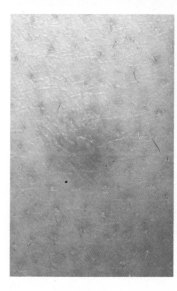

Early skin lesion in gonococcal septicaemia

PLATE 2

Sexually transmitted virus particles magnified 200 000 times

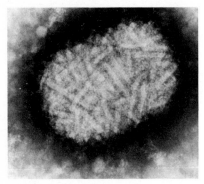

Molluscum contagiosum

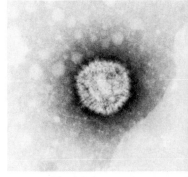

Cytomegalovirus

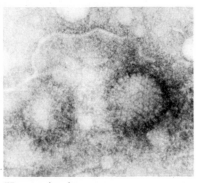

Herpes simplex

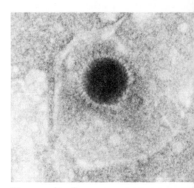

Herpes simplex

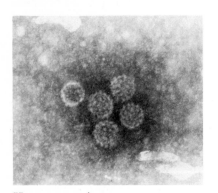

Human wart virus

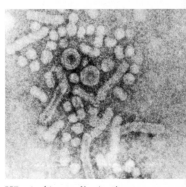

HB$_S$Ag/Australia Antigen
all at 200 000 ×   1 cm = 50 nm.

in any European country), the examining doctor can fill in a form which is then passed on to the police who will undertake a search. This is very rarely successful.

The Republic of Ireland. This is the only other country in the EEC, besides Great Britain, that recognizes venereology as a distinct specialty. So far, so good. Unfortunately there is only one full-time venereologist, who practises in Dublin, and elsewhere the sexually transmitted diseases are treated in clinics staffed by part-time clinicians. The figures are as unreliable as elsewhere − in 1976 there was not a single case of sexually transmitted disease reported from the county of Tipperary. In 1975 the figures for Ireland were 282 cases of gonorrhoea and 45 of syphilis. It is probable that many patients are treated privately and so these cases are not notified and also that some patients may come to England for diagnosis and treatment.

Specialist training in the Common Market countries

The minimum training period for a dermato-venereologist in the EEC is three years after qualification as a doctor. In some countries four years training is the norm; but only in Denmark, where two full years must be spent on the subject of the sexually transmitted diseases, is the subject given much weight. Since none of the countries have the separate specialty of venereology or genito-urinary medicine, the undergraduate teaching on these diseases is fragmented at best and may even be non-existent. The subject may be dealt with in passing by gynaecologists, urologists, and pathologists, but, in general, the newly qualified doctor will have had little cohesive training.

By contrast, in the United Kingdom venereology has to form part of the undergraduate medical curriculum and will be taught by a specialist venereologist or genito-urinary physician. After qualification, the recommendations of the Royal College of Physicians lay down that there should be three years of general training, including general medicine, neurology, and rheumatology, with, if possible, some ophthalmology, dermatology, and psychiatry, followed by *four* years of higher training in the specialty itself. A similar period of seven years is recommended for those intending to specialize in dermatology. There is thus quite a difference in the required training between Great Britain and the other members of the community.

4

Gonorrhoea

Gonorrhoea is the commonest venereal disease and the commonest *treatable* infection in the world today, with the exception, perhaps, of the non-specific genital infections. Gonorrhoea is not a modern disease, and it is probable that the reference in Leviticus, Chapter 15, to an 'issue out of flesh' is to gonococcal urethritis. Moses, in the following verses, gives advice about its infectivity and suggests a period of withdrawal from social intercourse during the infection. It is referred to by Hippocrates (300 BC), who regarded the penile discharge as a sign of impending cure of the disease. It was mentioned by many of the Greek philosophers and writers, including Aristotle, Plato, and Seneca, and eventually drove pleasure-loving Epicurus, who was plagued by gonococcal stricture, to suicide. It was Galen in the second century AD who invented the term gonorrhoea (from γονη = semen and ρεω = to flow), his view being that the discharge was an involuntary loss of sperm. Although Albert Neisser is credited with the discovery, in 1879, of the causative bacterium, *Neisseria gonorrhoeae*, which bears his name, seven years previously Hallier had noticed the presence of micro-organisms in the pus cells of gonococcal discharge.

There are several other bacteria similar to the gonococcus, which belong to the same family, the *Neisseriae*. The only other important one is *Neisseria meningitidis*, the usual cause of bacterial meningitis.

Gonorrhoea is an ubiquitous infection and is no respecter of social class or status. It affects males and females, young and old, heterosexuals and homosexuals, and shows no sign of diminution in prevalence despite world-wide control measures and the existence of effective antibiotic agents which can cure the disease once diagnosed.

There is much debate within the medical profession as to the infectivity of gonorrhoea. How likely is the disease to be passed on or aquired in any one given act of sexual intercourse between an infected and an uninfected person? There is no general agreement as to the answer to this question but the figure may lie somewhere between 50 and 80 per cent. The risk of catching the infection will obviously increase with the number of times intercourse takes place and will also depend on other factors, such as the sites that are infected and whether barrier contraceptives such as the condom are used.

Gonorrhoea is almost exclusively acquired sexually. That is to say, as a result of sexual intercourse or one of the variants of sexual behaviour, such as fellatio, cunnilingus, or rectal intercourse. Can it be caught from a lavatory seat? Well, the answer is that it can, but that, like other sexually transmitted diseases, this is an extremely rare method of transmission. If a lavatory seat is to be responsible then it is more likely to be the male who suffers. This is because the gonococcus rapidly perishes outside the human body, being dependent on the correct amount of warmth and moisture. It is possible for some urethral discharge from the penis to be transferred to the seat if the male is sitting down; and if a second male should accidentally touch the same part of the seat soon afterwards with his penis, then infection could be acquired. The gonococcus does not flourish on ordinary skin surfaces, preferring mucous membranes and internal tissues. It is therefore unlikely that a woman could either infect a lavatory seat or bring an infectable part of her anatomy in contact with such a seat.

The usual sites infected by the gonococcus are the urethra, throat, and rectum in the male, and the urethra, cervix, rectum, and throat in the female. Throat infection is more common among females who practice oral sex than among men, because the female's mouth is in direct contact with the infected part (the tip of the penis) whereas the male is in contact with an area not infected of its own right (the clitoris and vulva). Rectal infection in the male is usually the result of homosexual practice, such as anal or rectal intercourse, although infection can follow the use of stimulators such as vibrators or can occur as a result of insertion of a finger into the rectum during intercourse. The presence of infection in the female rectum, however, carries with it no such presumptions that the organism has been directly put there. Some 40 per cent of women with gonorrhoea are found to harbour the bug in the rectum and it is clear that in only a minority of cases has the gonococcus been 'placed' there. In the majority of cases, where intercourse has taken place in the 'missionary position' (woman lying on her back, man on top) the natural eversion of the anal mucous membrane during intercourse has brought this sensitive skin into contact with the moisture (in which the gonococcus can be found in quantity) produced by both male and female as a result of their sexual exertions.

Because of the natural apposition of penis and cervix during intercourse, in women the cervix is the site most commonly infected (about 90 per cent of cases). The urethra is the next most common site at 75 per cent, then the rectum (40 per cent), and finally the throat, infected in some 6 per cent of cases. This latter figure rises to 15 per cent if only those who admit to oro-genital contact are included.

Sexually Transmitted Diseases

The two important exceptions to the normal sexual method of transmission are in the case of young pre-pubertal girls and in newborn infants. Before girls reach puberty, the vulva and vagina have a different hormonal content and acidity, and the gonococcus can flourish in these areas. These young girls (and they are usually pre-teenagers) can catch gonorrhoea from infected materials, such as towels or flannels. If the young daughters of women with gonorrhoea are examined some 5 per cent will be found to be suffering from a gonococcal vulvo-vaginitis. They will either complain of nothing at all or perhaps of vulval soreness and a nasty discharge in that area. More often, however, a discharge will have been noticed in the underwear. It must not be forgotten, however, that gonorrhoea in young boys and girls can also be acquired sexually, and there are on record cases of boys and girls as young as five years old who have caught the infection in this way. The second non-sexual mode of transmission occurs at the time of childbirth. If the mother is suffering from untreated gonorrhoea involving the cervix at the time of birth, then the baby will come into contact with secretions containing gonococci in its passage through the birth canal. The organism may infect the eye of the infant with a resulting 'sticky eye', which usually develops within 48 hours. The eye becomes red and inflamed and there is a discharge of pus from between the lids. If treatment is not given, then the outer layer of the eye will be involved and scarring may occur. Damage to vision is then quite likely. This type of neonatal eye infection used to be the commonest cause of childhood blindness, but is now comparatively rare in civilized countries. Less than 5 per cent of sticky eyes in newborn babies are caused by the gonococcus in the United Kingdom at the present time, although it is more common in other parts of the world.

For the same reasons that the female is more likely to acquire infection in the throat than her male sexual partner, the homosexual male who practises oral sex is more likely to be infected in the throat than his heterosexual equivalent.

Whether or not normal mouth-to-mouth contact can spread gonorrhoea to an uninfected person is obviously an important question. There are certainly cases where this would seem to have been the only possible method of transmission, but the extent of the risk is hard to quantify. It would probably be true to say, however, that the long and passionate 'french' kiss is more likely to give the gonococcus a chance to spread than the toothless peck on the cheek from an aged aunt.

In men the signs and symptoms of gonorrhoea will appear after the incubation period, which is generally accepted as being between two and ten days. The majority of men who develop gonorrhoea in the penile urethra will notice two main symptoms. These are urethral discharge and discomfort passing urine (dysuria). There are several different causes of such symptoms in the male, but the development of either symptom in a sexually active person must be considered as most probably being due to a sexually transmitted disease. That is not to say that there are not many other 'innocent' causes for these two symptoms, but simply that urethritis, which is usually sexually transmitted, makes up the great majority of such cases. The usual differential diagnosis lies between non-specific urethritis and gonorrhoea. Although the discharge of either may vary from a barely discernible mucus to a gross, thick, profuse, and purulent exudate, the discharge of non-specific infection is usually lighter in texture, quantity, and colour. Both will often stain the underwear, but it is the gonococcal discharge that leaves a thick, yellow, encrusted deposit. Equally, the discomfort associated with gonorrhoea is usually of a greater order, and men who have suffered repeated attacks of both infections can usually tell which infection it is that they have on any given occasion. The discomfort in uncomplicated male gonorrhoea is made up of two components. There is the feeling of 'dis-ease' inside the penis due to inflammation of the urethra, which is aggravated by passing urine, and there is the discomfort which is felt at the tip of the penis, which is a manifestation of the inflammation at the urethral meatus. The observers of gonorrhoea in the days before effective treatment was available vividly described the symptoms of acute gonococcal urethritis. Thus the early discomfort is described by one author as 'a sensation of tingling or pricking which comes and goes suddenly, as if a fly were settling down'. This is followed by the inevitable pain on micturition described as passing 'a red-hot iron' or 'pieces of broken glass' or, by one patient, as if he had 'razors in his pipe'. The French had their own name for it — *chaudepisse*.

Nowadays the urinary symptoms seem to be of a lesser order. Maybe modern man is more stoical of nature, or perhaps, and this is more likely, there has been a real change in the symptom-producing capabilities of the gonococcus. The gonococcus has to adapt to any changes in its environment, particularly those which may compromise its chances of survival. Because the small one-celled bacteria have a rapid reproductive rate — they may divide every five minutes — evolution can take place over a much shorter time-scale than in larger organisms. Natural selection would favour those strains which produced a symptomless infection. Before the advent of bactericidal therapy no penalty to survival would be related to the production or not of symptoms. Since the last war, however, strains of the gonococcus which produce fewer symptoms will have had a greater chance of being passed on before treatment could be instituted. In the United States reports have suggested that up to 50 per cent of cases of gonorrhoea in males may be symptomless. Although this is an extreme figure, there is no doubt that completely symptomless infection in the male is becoming more common, and

33

those who do complain of symptoms seem to suffer considerably less than their pre-antibiotic forebears.

In the *female* a different set of rules applies. The gonococcus, a micro-biological master of male chauvanism, not only gives virtually no clues as to its presence in an infected female, but, should she attend a clinic or specialist for the purposes of diagnosis, it will only reveal itself in some 50 per cent of cases at the first visit compared to well over 90 per cent of cases in males. In the United Kingdom over 95 per cent of males with acute, uncomplicated gonorrhoea will develop symptoms of some sort. In contrast 50 per cent of women with acute gonorrhoea will have *no symptoms at all*. The remaining 50 per cent will develop symptoms, but these are of a non-specific nature. Thus 40 per cent will develop a degree of vaginal discharge. This would be a useful feature if it were not for the fact that a certain amount of vaginal discharge is perfectly normal and natural for a woman in her reproductive years; and what is more, this natural discharge is subject to a fair amount of variation depending on the stage of the menstrual cycle. In addition, there are many other infections, some sexually transmitted but many not, which also produce an alteration in the quantity or quality of the normal vaginal discharge. Are there any features which characterize the vaginal discharge that occurs with gonorrhoea? Sadly, the answer is no. The only feature in common with all the discharges associated with gonorrhoea is that they represent an alteration from the normal. One survey of the nature of the vaginal discharge in gonorrhoea demonstrated the wide spectrum covered. The most common description 'white' which occurred in 25 per cent of cases. Next came 'green' and 'yellow', 15 per cent each, and there then followed a host of pastel shades and textures running the gamut of 'grey' to 'gruesome' and 'florid' to 'foul'.

One in eight women with uncomplicated gonorrhoea will notice a degree of dysuria. This discomfort on passing urine can be related directly to the gonococcal infection, but again like the vaginal discharge, there are no distinguishing features to give clues that the gonococcus is responsible. Because three-quarters of women with gonorrhoea will have the infection in the urethra, one might expect urethral discharge to be a common finding in infected women. A discharge from the urethra can sometimes be demonstrated during the medical examination, but, since the urethral opening in the female is hidden between the folds of the labia, such a discharge will not be apparent to the woman herself; even if she examines herself, the natural moistness of this part of the body will tend to mask any contribution from the urethra. Unlike the dysuria associated with cystitis or upper renal tract infection, gonococcal dysuria is rarely combined with frequency of micturition. If frequency is present, it occurs usually only during the day and not at night. The other symptoms that may give clues to the presence of gonococcal infection in the woman are mostly produced when complications, such as involvement of the fallopian tubes, have set in. Rectal discharge may occur rarely as a result of infection of the back passage, but again infection of this site is usually asymptomatic.

This lack of symptoms in the female is one of the main reasons for the continuing endemic levels of gonorrhoea in the community. It also means that the infectious period, roughly estimated in the male as up to ten days, on average, is considerably longer in the female. There are several factors which help to prolong this period to perhaps three or four times that in the male. Assuming that she is asymptomatic, she either depends on the male who infected her to inform her of the diagnosis or, if he does not, wait for the next person with whom she has intercourse to develop symptoms, discover the diagnosis, and then contact her with the bad news. One estimate of this period puts it at about thirty days. During this time she is potentially infectious and any new sexual partners will run the risk of catching the infection.

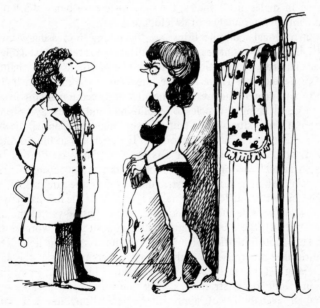

'Not only did my best friend not tell me, but it was her boy-friend who gave it me.'

There have been cases reported of gonorrhoea being passed on within four or five hours of its having been acquired, so, unlike the case with syphilis, there is no 'safe' period between catching and giving the infection. Because of this prolonged infectious period, the woman's contribution to the infected population is potentially much greater than the man's.

Complications

The problems that may occur if gonorrhoea is left untreated can usefully be divided into those that occur locally, that is, close to the original site of infection, and those that are systemic, due to dissemination of the infection (usually by means of the blood-stream) thoughout the body. Unlike many bacteria, the gonococcus has little capacity to 'eat away' at the tissue it infects. Usually, it simply colonizes the outer surface of the epithelium that it infects. If it comes across any orifices, holes, crypts, or glands, it will, however, gladly occupy these, and there may then be a degree of tissue destruction. The local complications of gonococcal infection can then be predicted from a knowledge of the local anatomy, with appropriate allowance being made for the differences between the sexes. The systemic complications are basically the same in males and females, the only difference being the female's considerably greater chance of developing them.

In men, local complications are becoming increasingly rare in industrialized rich countries, where medical care is readily available and the vast majority of infections are treated before there is any chance of problems developing. There may be infection in the many small glands found in and around the urethra. The infection occasionally involves the prostate gland, seminal vesicles, or epididymes and testes. Symptoms of infection at these sites will be pain and swelling with eventual discharge of pus if treatment is not forthcoming. If the glands in the urethra are involved, and chronic infection sets in, there may be fibrous tissue deposited at the sites of the chronic infection, and stricture formation may occur. When gonococcal stricture involves the urethra, there is obstruction to the outflow of urine, and, instead of the normal powerful stream (sometimes defined as adequate if the opposite wall of the urinal can be reached), there is a meagre dribble at best, and at worst nothing at all. This acute retention of urine constitutes one of medicine's most uncomfortable emergencies, with its habit of coming on at the end of and evening's drinking (usually beer) adding a bloated urgency to the situation. Gonococcal stricture is very rare these days, because of the widespread availability of appropriate medication, and it is largely elderly patients who attend a 'sounds' clinic, where the strictures can be dilated by means of metal, plastic, or gum instruments. Involvement of the spermatic cord, epididymis, or testis by infection can lead to sterility, but, again, this complication was much more common before the last World War and is rarely seen today.

In women, as in men, the local complications depend on the anatomy of the region, and, with one exception, these complications have

36

nuisance-value only. There may be infection in the glands of the urethra or labia. Bartholin's glands, which produce a secretion to aid lubrication during sexual intercourse, become extremely painful if infected. Before the 1940s over 50 per cent of Bartholin's gland infections were gonococcal in origin compared with less than 10 per cent today. The important exception is the involvement of the fallopian tubes and ovaries by the infective process. If infection is present for long in these organs then fertility may be seriously compromised. The fallopian tubes are exceedingly delicate organs lined by ciliated (hairy) epithelium, which can gently waft the ovum from the ovary to the uterus, where, if it has been fertilized, it will implant and become a developing foetus. As soon as the delicate lining has been interfered with, the ovum finds it difficult to make its way to the uterus and may either arrive too late for successful implantation or, which is worse, may implant in the tube itself, giving rise to an ectopic pregnancy (tubal pregnancy). Quite apart from the problems of decreased fertility and the dangers of ectopic pregnancy, the chronic ill-health and malaise which often follow infection of the tubes make this complication one to be avoided at all costs. The danger time for development of tubal complications with gonorrhoea is the menstrual period. It has been shown that during the period there is flow of menstrual products backwards up the fallopian tubes and even into the abdominal cavity. It is this retrograde flow that is probably responsible for the spread of infection internally. It is at this point that gonorrhoea may start to produce symptoms in the female. She may develop lower abdominal pain often on one side only (and often, if it is on the right side, confused with acute appendicitis), backache, and fever. She may notice that the menstrual period is heavier than usual and there may be some deep dyspareunia and dysmenorhoea. If the infection is unchecked, peritonitis may follow and gonorrhoea becomes a life-threatening emergency. In this country between 5 and 10 per cent of cases of gonorrhoea in women go on to develop a degree of tubal involvement, and only a few of these will lead to peritonitis. Infection of the fallopian tubes must remain the most important cause of infertility today, although only a minority of cases will be due to gonorrhoea.

Systemic complications occur in between 1 and 2 per cent of cases of gonorrhoea and are less common in men than in women in a ratio of about one to four. These complications are only likely to set in if the infection has been present for some time, and this is only likely to happen if the infection is an asymptomatic one. The infection is usually blood-borne and may infect almost any organ in the body. The most common sites for infection are the joints and the skin. The heart may be involved in a gonococcal myocarditis, pericarditis, or endocarditis. The nervous system may be involved and a meningitis produced, similar to that produced by the meningococcus, or the liver may be affected. But, once again, these complications are comparatively rare, and, these days, fairly easy to treat. In the days before effective treatment, endocarditis, in which the valves of the heart are themselves affected, was a very serious complication, a measure of which is given by the title of a contemporary report: 'Gonococcal endocarditis – a report of twelve cases, *with ten post-mortem examinations*' (my italics). When this complication does occur these days (and the only reports are from the United States) it may necessitate open-heart surgery for the replacement of the defective valve.

Diagnosis

Although in some cases gonorrhoea may be suspected from the symptoms or signs of the disease, in the final analysis the diagnosis hangs on the identification of the gonococcus, either directly in a sample of mucus or other material from an infected site by microscopic examination, or by its growth in the laboratory after inoculation of such material on appropriate culture media. If a man is suspected of having gonorrhoea, examination of the discharge from his urethra will demonstrate the organism in over 90 per cent of the cases when it is there. A sample is taken and placed on a microscope slide and stained with coloured dyes which show up different structures in varying colours and shades. A satisfactory system for staining the majority of bacteria uses Gram's method (named after its inventor). With this method some structures take on a purple coloration while others take up the red counter-stain. Most bacteria come into the category either of Gram-positive, which take up the purple stain, or Gram-negative which don't. The neisseria are all Gram-negative organisms. The white cells from the blood, the polymorphonuclear leucocytes or 'pus cells', which are responsible for scavenging and consuming unwelcome intruders in the body, can be seen to have phagocytosed, or eaten, the bacteria, which thus become 'intracellular'. With the final diagnostic criterion that depends on the gonococcus's propensity for going round in pairs as 'diplococci' we have the microscopic finding that enables the diagnosis to be made in cases of suspected gonorrhoea – *Gram-negative intracellular diplococci*. The diagnosis of gonorrhoea in man can thus be confirmed in the majority of cases within the time it takes to stain and examine a slide of urethral discharge from the penis – a matter of some fifteen or twenty minutes.

With women, even allowing for the fact that slides of material from three sites, urethra, cervix, and rectum may be examined, this early diagnosis is only possible in about 50 per cent of cases. That is not to suggest that the gonococcus is not present at these different sites but that it is difficult to identify microscopically. To make the diagnosis, therefore, it is necessary to rely on the laboratory's ability to grow the bacterium, and this culture process demands particular care and expertise. The gonococcus is a fastidious organism and demands not only the normal foodstuffs found in bacterial growth media (normally blood products, meat extract, or 'chocolate', which is boiled blood) but it relies on the correct temperature, humidity, and carbon dioxide content in the surrounding atmosphere. With all this it is rather slow to grow and frequently when the culture plate is examined for evidence of gonococcal growth it will be found to be overgrown by other bacteria or yeasts, making it difficult or impossible to identify the gonococcus. Most modern culture media contain both antibiotics and anti-fungal agents to which the gonococcus is not sensitive, to inhibit the growth of competitive organisms.

It is important that all the possibly infected sites are sampled, since in a small percentage of cases of gonorrhoea the rectum or urethra may be the only site involved. This occurs in about five per cent of cases of gonorrhoea for either site. It is also important to examine the throat for the presence of gonococci (by cultural methods), since, not only may it be the only site involved, but it is rather more difficult to eradicate the infection from this place.

Case history. Mrs Gladys H., a 37-year-old, separated, sweet-shop owner in a south-coast holiday resort was named as a contact by a young man with gonorrhoea. He had gone further and had suggested that he had actually caught the disease from her. She was considerably upset by this and amongst protestations of sexual continence said that, apart from this young man, she had not had intercourse with anybody else since her husband, who had left her ten months previously. On examination there was little abnormal to see, the cervix looked very healthy and there was no excess of vaginal discharge. Both slides and cultures from the cervix and urethra were negative for gonorrhoea and were duly repeated. The results of the second set of tests again turned out to be negative and she refused any further investigation.

The incident was forgotten until the young man returned to the clinic five months later with a second attack of gonorrhoea. He was 'effing and blinding' because he said that he had caught the infection from Mrs H. again. With a certain reluctance she agreed to have a further examination, and tests were taken from the cervix and urethra. These all turned out to be negative and the examining doctor decided to take rectal samples when she returned for her results as he felt she would be unlikely to come back a third time. Both the microscope slide and the culture were positive for the gonococcus. Although the young man and Mrs H. denied rectal intercourse, it is probable that this was the site that had served as a source of the infection, which had presumably originated with her husband over a year previously.

When the problems associated with the microscopic diagnosis, particularly in women, are coupled with the difficulties in the 'horticultural' aspects of the gonococcus, and these are both combined with the reluctance of specialists in certain countries to examine material from potentially infected patients, it is not surprising that the reported rates for gonorrhoea from some areas are absurdly low. Where there exists such a reluctance to carry out the correct diagnostic procedures or, as is often the case, there is simply a dearth of properly trained specialists, the natural result is treatment without diagnosis, the haphazard use of antibiotics (such as penicillin for all urethral discharges), and an increase in antibiotic resistance of the gonococci coupled with an infuriating denial of the problem, 'Just look at our figures. We have no problem with gonorrhoea in this part of the world'.

Treatment

The treatment of gonorrhoea was transformed by the discovery of the chemotherapeutic agents – the sulphonamides – before the Second World War. This was followed soon after by penicillin and then a host of other antibiotics, very many of which are or were effective in the treatment of gonorrhoea. In 1937 there came the first medical report in the *Journal of the American Medical Association* of the successful use of the sulphonamides in the treatment of acute gonorrhoea. The treatments that were thus superseded have been touched upon in Chapter 2, but suffice it to say that there was general and unqualified relief from both doctors and patients that they had passed. During the last years of the war it was noticed that rather a high proportion of soldiers were failing to be cured by the standard doses of M & B 693, as the sulphonamide was called, and this was the first clue to the potential in the gonococcus for developing resistance to antibiotics. Luckily penicillin became available and was found to be highly effective in what we would consider today to be almost homeopathic doses. A textbook of medicine published in 1953 recommends 200 000 units of penicillin as a treatment. Nowadays, between ten and twenty-five times as much penicillin would need to be given routinely with the addition of another drug, probenecid, which helps to maintain high blood- and tissue levels of the antibiotic by reducing the rate at which it is eliminated by the kidneys, and even then there is no guarantee of success.

This is because of the widespread development of partial resistance to penicillin and other antibiotics by the gonococcus, due to its evolution as a response to changes in its environment. This is a process which is going on all the time in the world of bacteria, and drug firms are managing to keep ahead, just, by producing newer (and inevitably, more expensive) antibiotics that will still be effective.

In spite of the development of partial resistance, penicillin is still the treatment of choice in gonorrhoea. The ideal treatment, irrespective of the antibiotic, is one which has its effect with a single dose. This may be an injection or, as is increasingly common, a number of tablets or capsules all to be taken at the same time. In this respect gonorrhoea differs from the majority of other bacterial infections, for which it has always been assumed that a *course* of treatment lasting several days or even weeks is needed.

A recent development with frightening implications is the isolation in several parts of the world of strains of gonococci which are not just partially resistant to penicillin, but can produce an enzyme, β-lactamase, which actually breaks down and neutralizes penicillin completely. If this gonococcus should become widespread, the problems of gonorrhoea control would be multiplied manyfold. There was an outbreak of infection with this organism in Liverpool in 1976, which was thankfully controlled by dint of exhaustive contact-tracing, and there have only been sporadic single cases since then, mostly imported from abroad.

In the treatment of gonorrhoea with complications, a longer course of antibiotic therapy is needed and this must usually be combined with a period of rest, preferably in bed, preferably alone.

5

Non-specific genital infection

If gonorrhoea is the commonest venereal disease, then non-specific infection is the commonest sexually transmitted disease — the difference being one of definition. Under this heading comes a variety of related conditions, probably with several causes. Non-specific urethritis (NSU), non-gonococcal urethritis (NGU), post-gonococcal urethritis (PGU), and non-specific genital infection (NSGI) all refer to genital conditions which have many of the characteristics of sexually transmitted diseases and yet defy accurate categorization in terms of their aetiology. The problem with these diseases is that they are diagnosed on the basis of *indirect* evidence of infection rather than by identifying a specific micro-organism. They thus occupy a rather special place in the spectrum of infectious human disease, since, without being able to find the germ responsible, it is not only rather difficult to be sure that the disease is present in the first place, but, having given a treatment for which there can be no definite evidence of efficacy, since no organism has been eliminated, it can be very difficult to tell whether the infection has resolved or even whether the patient is better. This barrenness of bacterial feedback coupled with many patients' understandable neurosis makes the condition one that provides difficulties for patient and doctor alike. The term 'non-specific' is unsatisfactory, although in common usage, because it lumps together those cases where a cause can be established with those in which no aetiological agent can be found.

Urethritis

Urethritis simply means inflammation of the urethra. It carries with it no assumptions about the cause and just describes the inflammatory process that is taking place in the epithelial lining inside the penis. The most important finding is a polymorphonuclear leucocyte response. These 'pus' cells migrate from the blood to sites of noxious stimuli, be they bacterial, fungal, viral, or inanimate. They do not in themselves betoken infection, although they can be taken as indirect evidence of infection in many cases. When a specific pathogenic organism is implicated, such as the gonococcus, there can be assumed a natural cause-and-effect, and the presence of pus-cells is easily explained. With non-gonococcal urethritis there may be an equal pus-cell response with the difference that there are no pathogenic organisms to be found under the microscope. It is generally assumed that pus-cells in the urethra are synonymous with infection and the pus-cell is treated vigorously from Bath to Bangkok and from Memphis to Madras as if it were an infectious organism itself. No doubt many, probably a majority, of the cases of non-gonococcal urethritis are due to infectious organisms, but there remains a hard core of cases from which no pathogenic germs can be isolated and for which it is just conceivable that antibiotic treatment may not be the best therapy. For all that, there are certain well-defined causes of urethritis and they will be dealt with first.

Causes of urethritis

Bacteria. Apart from gonococcal infection, certain other bacteria are sometimes found in the urethra and may be responsible for the signs and symptoms of NGU. The bacteria which are usually found in the intestine, such as *Escherichia coli*, when found in conjunction with urethritis, often indicate infection higher in the uro-genital tract. Thus, there may appear to be a urethritis when the main problem is in fact an infection in the bladder or in the kidneys, or, more locally, in the prostate gland.

Certain types of small bacteria, called mycoplasma or ureaplasma, have for a long time been thought to be responsible for some cases of NGU. The most recent evidence, however, indicates that, although mycoplasma are undoubtedly sexually transmitted, they are often present in the genital tract in a non-pathogenic or commensal capacity. Some strains may be responsible for a small percentage of non-gonococcal infections, but are often found in people who have neither symptoms nor any other evidence of urethritis.

Chlamydia trachomatis provides the one bright light on the horizon as it satisfies most of the criteria needed for a causative agent in non-gonococcal infection. We will return to it later.

Fungi. Candida albicans and related yeast-like fungi are commonly found in the genital tract, particularly in women, and do not often produce infection or symptoms in the male. When they do, it usually takes the form of a balanitis, inflammation of the glans penis under the foreskin. Occasionally the infection may involve the tip of the penis, just inside the urethral meatus. In these cases, there may be a 'terminal' urethritis mimicking the symptoms of a non-specific urethritis.

Viruses. Herpes simplex, the virus responsible for cold sores on the lips and face, is also involved in genital infection. The sores that it produces are usually found on the external surface of the penis in the male, but rarely the site of infection may be inside the urethra, and in these cases recurrent 'non-specific urethritis' may occur, which is particularly resistant to treatment. Viral cultures during an attack will give the diagnosis in cases such as these.

Chemicals. Any strong chemicals, if allowed to come into contact with the urethral mucous membrane, which is very sensitive, may set up an irritative urethritis. The pre-antibiotic irrigations used organic silver solutions, mercuric salts, potassium permanganate, and even, by a very sporting Dr Porosz of Budapest during the last century, nitric acid. Solutions of these chemicals were often run into the urethra under considerable pressure and were accepted, by their proponents, as producing a urethritis themselves as part of their cure. These days there may be a reaction to the chemicals in some of the modern spermicides and vaginal products on the market. The rash application of strong antiseptic solutions to prevent or ward off infection is another rare cause of urethritis.

Protozoa. Trichomonas vaginalis is undoubtedly a cause of non-gonococcal urethritis but is not the elusive 'organism x' that has been sought so exhaustively. Male contacts of women with trichomonal vaginitis can be shown to harbour the organism in a certain proportion of cases, and this proportion can be increased if extra care and time is taken looking for the protozoon. This includes massaging the prostate gland and massaging the urethra over a metal sound. By this means, twice as many cases of trichomonal urethritis can be found among these male contacts. The fact that this extra testing can produce extra diagnoses implies that a proportion of those cases diagnosed as NGU would turn out to be trichomonal if only the organism were adequately looked for. This is certainly true, but this explanation might only account for some 4 or 5 per cent or NGU cases. It is likely that *T. vaginalis* is not at its happiest in the male urethra, and providing exposure to the protozoon does not again occur during this period, in about a week most men will probably eliminate the organism from the urethra without the aid of treatment. Since in women it is a largely vaginal infection, the advantages given to the man of washing out the urethra with urine several times a day do not apply. If a man is to infect a women with *Trichomonas vaginalis*, this is most likely to occur if he has intercourse with her fairly soon after he himself has acquired the infection.

Foreign bodies. This quaint description is not a manifestation of that well-known British chauvanism and insularity, but refers to an odd habit the human animal has of inserting bits and pieces of various shapes and sizes into different holes and orifices. Women may insert articles into their vaginas for purposes of masturbation, and men will insert articles

44

into their urethras with the same intention. If the object is not removed, it can act as a focus of infection and, in the case of the male, may produce a urethritis which will be resistant to treatment until the offending article has been removed.

Case history. Freddie P., a 53 year-old, single accountant presented in the casualty department of a local hospital complaining that, for the last four days, he had noticed beads of pus at the tip of his penis when he woke up in the morning. He had also felt a stinging sensation every time he passed urine. On examination there was a thick discharge visible at the urethral meatus. Further examination revealed a hard swelling at the base of the penis and the question of a foreign body was raised with Mr P. He strongly denied inserting anything into his urethra and so an X-ray was taken. It showed a radiopaque object, which was at first difficult to identify. When presented with the X-ray, Mr P. explained all. It seemed that he used a safety-pin inserted into the urethra for the purposes of masturbation and, in order that it should not be lost, he tied a length of cotton to it. One day the inevitable happened and the cotton broke. Instead of relaxing and letting nature take its course – it would probably have passed quite easily when he passed his water – he panicked and tried to remove the safety pin by not so gentle manipulations from the outside. Not surprisingly the safety-pin opened under this onslaught and landed Mr P in a painful and difficult situation which needed the ministrations of a surgeon to sort out.

The variety of foreign bodies found in and around the genitalia is enormous, but, like the previously mentioned causes of urethritis, they make up but a small proportion of the cases of urethritis.

In total, the above causes account for, perhaps, 10 per cent of all cases of 'NSU'.

Chlamydia trachomatis. The remaining 90 per cent of cases remained an obstinate mystery until the middle fifties, when it became possible to culture this obscure organism on the yolk-sac of the chicken embryo. Since then a great deal has been learnt about its role in the pathogenesis of non-specific genital infection. The reason for chlamydia's comparatively late arrival on the microbiological scene is that, although behaving in many ways like a virus, it is in fact a highly specialized and adapted bacterium. Thus, although it is amenable to antibiotic therapy like a bacterium, it is, like a virus, an obligatory intracellular parasite. This means that it depends on the host's cells' own energy-producing system to provide for its own growth and reproduction. It was this particular feature that made its isolation so difficult, for it is impossible to grow chlamydia on the normal media used for bacteria, since they do not contain living cells. The existence of this group of organisms was first suspected by two unpronouncable German scientists in 1907, who gave their names to the Halberstaedter-Prowazek bodies seen inside ocular cells infected by the agent which causes trachoma. It is now recognized that the trachoma agent is very closely related to the organism that causes non-specific urethritis and is responsible for 50 per cent of sticky eyes in newborn babies and for a proportion of cases of salpingitis in women.

The genus *Chlamydia* is divided into two main groups. The type-B chlamydiae are animal pathogens, and the only important member as far as human infection is concerned is that which affects birds and causes pigeon-fancier's lung or psittacosis.

The type-A chlamydiae include the sub-groups responsible for trachoma, non-specific infection, and lympho-granuloma venereum. The major step forward in understanding the role of chlamydia in oculo-genital infection came in the early sixties when a group of workers in London published several reports connecting eye infection in the newborn baby with the presence of chlamydia in the mother's genital tract and non-specific urethritis in the father. Chlamydial infection was thus shown to have similarities to gonorrhoea in this respect. It was shown that the organism could cause conjunctivitis in baboons and, after inoculation in the urethra, a urethritis as well. Re-isolation from the baboon showed the organism to be the same one as that originally isolated from a baby's sticky eye. Further work from many parts of the world have demonstrated chlamydia in a proportion of patients with non-gonococcal infection and, when they have been tested, in their sexual partners. There is general agreement that *Chlamydia trachomatis* is the pathogen responsible for a high percentage of cases of NSU, but the best isolation rates still remain below 70 per cent of cases and are more usually in the region of 40 to 50 per cent. There still remains a variable minority of cases of non-gonococcal urethritis which are due neither to chlamydial infection nor to one of the other causes mentioned earlier.

It is these cases, where no pathogen can be isolated yet there are pus cells to be found in the urethra, that major problems of diagnosis arise. In practice the situation is worse than described. Because of the difficulty in isolating *C. trachomatis*, the time it takes to do so, and the expense involved, there are very few laboratories prepared to take on routine chlamydia isolation. At present there are less than ten laboratories in Britain that can isolate the organism, and most of these are working as research units rather than as service units prepared to isolate chlamydia as part of the standard diagnostic screening that should be available. Although there are laboratories in Europe and the United States that can grow chlamydia, again they are working as research rather than service units. It can be calculated that during 1979, 18 000 women will attend clinics in England suffering from chlamydial infection, which they have no hope of getting diagnosed and therefore treated. These women are at risk of developing salpingitis, of giving birth to babies with eye infections and of passing the infection on to their sexual partner in the form of NSU.

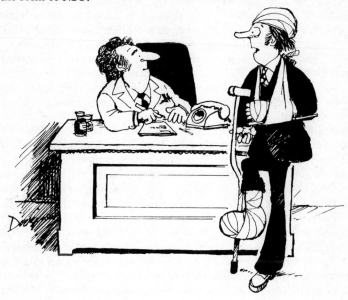

'I did it falling off a lavatory seat.'

It can be seen, then, that we are dealing with a condition that is some two or three times as common as gonorrhoea, for which an organism is implicated and can be grown in perhaps 50 per cent of cases; and yet there are no facilities, generally, for its isolation. As far as the male is concerned, this might not matter too much were it not for the fact that some of these cases of NSU or 'pus cells in the urethra' may very well not be manifestations of infection. It might be thought reasonable to treat all cases of NSU so diagnosed when they initially present to the clinic as if they had a sexually transmitted disease and prescribe appropriate antibiotics, and, indeed, this is common practice in most clinics. Where the difficulty arises is in cases of so-called 'relapse'. If a patient returns after a prolonged course of antibiotic therapy and is still found to be harbouring the ubiquitous pus cell in the urethra, then it may well be that he has reinfected himself from his, as yet untreated, sexual partner. It is also possible, though unlikely, that the prolonged course of treatment was inadequate to eliminate the organism responsible. It is even possible (and I suspect that many 'relapses' fall into this category) that the pus cells do not represent active infection and are a residual sign of past or resolving infection. If a parallel is taken with the treatment of another infection, say, lobar pneumonia, at the end of a ten-day course of penicillin treatment, there will be no sign of the responsible bacteria and, if the antibiotics are stopped, the bacteria will not return and reinfect the lung. However, the patient is likely to continue coughing for some time after the antibiotics have been stopped, and the sputum that is produced when the patient coughs will be found to contain numerous pus cells on microscopic examination. Nobody would claim that these pus cells are evidence of continuing infection, rather that they are evidence of resolving *inflammation* and as such are not appropriately treated with antibiotics.

It will have been gathered from what has gone before that the non-gonococcal infections are considerably less easy both to diagnose and to treat than gonorrhoea itself. This difficulty is compounded by three further factors: the slightness of the symptoms in the majority of cases, the length of treatment, and the difficulty in assessing cure. It has been postulated that the symptoms of gonorrhoea have diminished since the introduction of effective antibiotic therapy. It may well be that this reduction in severity of symptoms has brought the symptoms of NSU much closer to those of gonorrhoea and thereby exaggerated their importance. In the eighteenth century Boswell describes his attack of gonorrhoea, which is complicated by an attack of epididymo-orchitis, and, after a miserable six weeks of self-imposed confinement at home, rejoices that he is cured because all he can see is a slight 'gleet' which he is happy to ignore. I have no doubt that he would have been diagnosed as NSU today and treated accordingly. Boswell certainly did not consider that it merited more than a brief mention, and was in no way put out by it.

The symptoms of NGU in the man are similar to those of gonococcal urethritis, but less severe. Dysuria and urethral discharge are the main presenting symptoms, appearing anything from one to six weeks after catching the infection, with the majority occurring at two or three weeks. The discharge is usually less profuse than a gonococcal one, often being described as a 'feeling of dampness' rather than a full-blown urethral discharge. Although it can be as profuse as a gonococcal discharge, it is sometimes only seen first thing in the morning before urine has been passed. The discharge is not as thick as a gonococcal one and is more often mucoid and clear in colour. The dysuria is also of a lesser order described as 'tingling' rather than 'burning' during micturition. There may be some staining of underwear, again less than that found with gonorrhoea.

As with gonorrhoea, non-gonococcal infection in the female does not produce signs or symptoms that enable it to be diagnosed clinically. There may be evidence of a urethritis in the female, but it is more common for there to be a cervicitis. This is unlikely to produce anything

48

more than a slight increase in vaginal discharge which has no particular distinguishing features. Because cervicitis, cervical erosions, and discharges are so common in sexually active women, none of these features help more than indirectly with the diagnosis. This means that the woman is crippled as far as the diagnosis of non-gonococcal infection is concerned. At least with the man, a urethritis can be diagnosed, albeit imperfectly, by noticing pus cells in the urethra, but the same criteria cannot be applied to the woman. One is left with either diagnosing non-specific genital infection in all the female sexual partners of men with NSU or hoping that facilities for chlamydia isolation become widely available in the near future.

The medical profession is divided as to whether female NSU-contacts should be treated. Probably a majority would recommend treatment of the female sexual partner(s) with at least the first attack of NSU, but, as with gonorrhoea where up to one third of female gonorrhoea contacts can be shown not to have the disease, such a policy of treatment without diagnosis is bound to lead to a certain amount of overtreatment.

Complications

The local complications occurring with non-gonococcal infection are similar to those with gonorrhoea and are equally rare. In the male, infection may spread to urethral glands and the prostate. The seminal vesicles can become infected and inflamed, as may the epididymis and testis. In the female the glands of the labia may be involved by infection, and the process may spread upwards to involve the fallopian tubes with acute or chronic non-gonococcal salpingitis.

A rare but important complication of non-gonococcal urethritis is Reiter's disease or syndrome. This is a systemic condition which superficially resembles the problems associated with disseminated gonococcal infection in that the joints and skin are involved. That is as far as the resemblance goes, however, for the pattern of joint and skin involvement in the two conditions is very different and in addition other systems are involved in Reiter's disease which are spared in gonococcal dermatitis and arthritis. The important difference between the two conditions is in the nature of the systemic complications. In the case of gonorrhoea, the complications are a direct result of bacteria spreading through the body. Thus, the bacterium can be found in affected joints, or in the skin lesions, or in the bloodstream and any ill-effects can be directly ascribed to the activity of the bacteria. With Reiter's disease the ill-effects are due to the body's reaction rather than to actual infection. Some people are more likely to develop these complications and can be identified by demonstrating the presence of a particular tissue-type in their body make-up. This process, a little like blood-grouping, is used to match tissues from a donor with the tissues of a prospective patient who is waiting for a kidney transplant. A high proportion of patients who develop Reiter's disease can be shown to have HLA B27 tissue antigen which is also found in people who develop arthritis associated with the skin disease psoriases and those with ankylosing spondylitis. It appears that certain people have a predisposition to develop Reiter's disease and it is possible that the organism responsible for NGU can act as a 'trigger' which sets off the inflammatory process.

Although Reiter's disease usually follows NGU in this country, in other parts of the world it is well recognized as following certain forms of dysentery. In these cases there is a quite typical urethritis, even though there is no question of the urethra being the primary site of infection, and no organisms can be recognized or cultured from this site.

The most common joints involved in Reiter's disease are those of the lower limb, particularly around the ankle. There may be small ulcers on the penis and in the mouth and in some cases the condition also affects the eyes. Rarely the valves of the heart can be involved. It should be stressed that this complication is rare, and only a minority of cases go on to develop long-term problems. This syndrome is much more common among males.

The final and perhaps most important complication of non-specific infection is one that is more often iatrogenic (doctor-induced) in origin. Because of the uncertainty about the diagnosis, the prolonged treatment often advocated, and the slightness of the symptoms in many cases, it is often very difficult to persuade patients that they are cured. Many people get it into their minds that it is a serious condition and restrictions on sexual activity, the forbidding of alcohol, and prolonged treatment do nothing to dispel this mistaken belief. It is not surprising that NSU neurosis occurs in many cases. Once a patient has convinced himself that he has still got NSU, it is very difficult to persuade him that all the symptoms he complains of are in fact perfectly normal.

Treatment

Although many antibiotics are used to treat non-gonococcal urethritis, the most popular are the tetracyclines, which seem to have the best therapeutic effect and have the most powerful activity against chlamydia in the laboratory. Opinions vary as to how long antibiotic treatment should last, and periods differ between four and twenty-one days. It is impossible to define an optimal treatment period but it should obviously be long enough to eliminate the one main cause of non-specific infection, chlamydia. There is experimental work to show that a week or ten days may not be long enough and a fortnight to three weeks is probably the best theoretical period.

It has been one of the principle tenets of urethritis treatment policy that the patient should take no alcohol during the treatment period.

Non-specific genital infection

Whether this has any foundation in science or whether it reflects the old-fashioned 'punitive' approach, men up and down the country, known for their ten-pint capacity or love for fine wine, are receiving old-fashioned looks as they ask for a half-pint of lime juice or a tonic on its own. Although alcohol is undoubtedly excreted in the urine and could theoretically act as an inflammatory agent in a case of urethritis, it is probably enough to reduce alcohol intake rather than cut it out altogether — there have been no convincing scientific trials to show that alcohol consumption delays resolution of urethritis.

Treatment of non-specific infection in women is the same as for men, although some clinics do not believe that female contacts should be treated. It is usual to advise against further sexual intercourse until the treatment is finished.

Case history. Jonathon G., a 38-year-old single executive, did not regard himself as promiscuous and preferred a stable relationship to a series of 'one-night stands'. In spite of this he was sexually very experienced and attractive to women and found it difficult to turn down their advances. With a sexual history spanning more than twenty years and including fifty or sixty different partners, he regarded VD as something that happened to other people, and was somewhat surprised to develop a mild urethral discharge five weeks after first sleeping with his new girl-friend, Angela, who was younger than him and relatively sexually inexperienced. His last sexual encounter before meeting Angela had been four months previously and Angela had not slept with anyone for nine months since breaking up with her previous boy-friend with whom she had been going out for a year.

One week before attending the special clinic, Jonathon had noticed some staining of his underpants and on examining his penis, not a thing he was in the habit of doing, he found that he could express a little clear mucoid discharge from it. Now that his mind had been alerted, he examined himself several times a day and, when the discharge didn't go away, he decided to attend. He had also noticed that there was a slight discomfort when he passed urine. When examined in the clinic, the discharge was noted and after microscopy had confirmed the diagnosis of NGU, he was started on a three-week course of tetracycline. His new girl-friend was also examined and nothing abnormal was found, although she did say that there had been some increase in her vaginal discharge for some months. Although no bacteria could be isolated — culture for chlamydia was negative for both of them — she was given an equivalent three-week course of antibiotics. His urethral discharge and her vaginal discharge had both cleared by two weeks, and when they were seen one month after their original visit, there was no sign of infection or inflammation.

All was well for the next fortnight, then Jonathon phoned up to say that his infection had returned. At his insistence he was seen the same day, and exhaustive examination failed to reveal any abnormality. He

51

was still convinced that there was something wrong and said that he had noticed some urethral discharge first thing in the morning and also a slight 'tingle' when he first passed urine in the day. He had got into the habit of examining himself minutely every morning and would squeeze and 'milk' his urethra to see if there was any sign of discharge. When he found that he *could* demonstrate some discharge in the early mornings he was convinced that his infection had returned, not realizing that the majority of males can produce a certain amount of mucus at the urethral meatus in the morning if they try.

In this case a budding urethral neurosis was nipped before it could really blossom. Often, however, an attack of non-specific urethritis can be followed by months, if not years, of needless worry and anxiety, simply because, following the mind's focusing on the genitalia, the patient has noticed certain characteristics of his sexual organs for the first time, and normality has become abnormality.

6

Vaginal discharge

Vaginal discharge is one of the commonest female complaints and one that is in general poorly understood and looked after. Its causes are myriad, ranging from the benign to the bizarre, from the malignant to the mundane. It is a symptom which many women are too embarrassed to consult their doctors about, and which many doctors are too ignorant to do anything about. A certain amount of vaginal discharge is a normal and natural feature of a part of the body with several different if related functions. It has to provide an appropriate milieu for the sex act, to act as a channel for the menstrual flow, which is the shedding of the unused lining of the uterus when conception and implantation of the fertilized ovum has not taken place, and also furnish the route by which the baby exits.

The vagina, like the mouth, ears, or any other orifice open to the outside world is, as a matter of course, populated by many micro-organisms, most of which rarely cause problems and give their host little reason to be aware of their presence. There are several different relationships between bacteria and larger organisms: *symbiosis* is a relationship of mutual benefit to both the host and the micro-organism. An example is the presence of nitrogen-fixing bacteria in certain plants such as peas or beans. Neither would prosper without the help of the other. *Commensalism* is a relationship of mutual tolerance. The bacterium does no harm and indeed, as in the case of some bacteria in the gut, may, by making vitamins, actually benefit the host. *Pathogenicity* is the capacity of certain organisms to produce disease. Some pathogenic organisms may not manifest their disease-provoking properties in certain sites, where they may behave as commensals.

The preponderant bacterium in the adult vagina is the lactobacillus. This bacterium is unusual in that it tolerates extremely acid conditions. It converts glycogen, a form of carbohydrate, to lactic acid, which most other micro-organisms are unable to tolerate. Lactobacilli are the organisms responsible for the souring of milk, and yoghurt is one of the end-products of this bacterium's effect on milk. As long as there is a healthy collection of lactobacilli in the vagina, conditions will be un-favourable for other micro-organisms, and, although a few such organisms

53

may be isolated, their presence does not signify any important infection.

Viral infections may also cause a change or increase in vaginal discharge. *Herpes simplex* infection, when it involves the cervix, can cause a profuse discharge. Even measles sometimes produces a vaginal discharge.

When most people refer to a 'vaginal' discharge, they are, in fact, begging the question of the source of their complaint. What they mean is a discharge visible at the entrance to the vagina. The distinction is quite important, for there are certain truly 'vaginal' infections in which the actual surface of the vagina is involved in the infective process and there are infections of the cervix and uterus which may also cause a discharge that appears 'vaginal' but is, in fact, cervical or uterine in origin. Thus, the vaginal discharge associated with gonorrhoea in women really reflects cervical rather than vaginal infection.

Candida albicans

In departments of genito-urinary medicine, the commonest pathogen isolated from attending women is *Candida albicans*. This yeast-like fungus is an ubiquitous organism which is found as a commensal in up to 70 per cent of people's intestines. It causes 'thrush', which is an infection of mucous membranes occurring from time to time in young children, characterized by white patches developing in the mouth. It also causes a vulvitis and vaginitis in women and a balanitis in men. In some people whose immunological defences are weakened, either by the effect of drugs, cancer, or as a result of a congenital defect in antibody production, the fungus can invade the external skin surface, which is resistant to such infection under normal circumstances. In certain serious blood disorders it can invade other parts of the body, such as the lungs or central nervous system, with severe, if not fatal, consequences. In normal circumstances, however, an easy truce prevails with candida giving no symptoms from its home in the bowel and man therefore using no drugs in an attempt to eliminate it.

The close proximity of the entrance of the vagina to the anus makes the anus a particular threat to the vagina as a source of candida and provides the bacteria to infect the bladder in cases of cystitis. A few colonies of the fungus can often be grown from the vagina of a completely healthy and symptom-free woman. The presence of a few colonies of candida does not constitute infection, however, any more than the presence of many other organisms in small numbers in the vagina means that they are there in a pathogenic capacity. A delicate balance is kept in the microbiological eco-system of the vagina in health, with the lactobacillus being the predominant organism, and others being kept at bay by the very acid environment that this bacterium produces. If, for some reason, the lactobacillus is no longer present in the vagina, other organisms take advantage of the opportunity and invade.

Vaginal discharge

The worst offenders in this modern age are the 'broad-spectrum' antibiotics. These exercise their antimicrobial powers against a wide variety of different bacteria and when given for, say, a sore throat, will also kill off many of the normal commensal organisms in the intestine (which is why a lot of people develop diarrhoea when taking antibiotics), and will also destroy the normal bacterial flora in the vagina. Since candida is not a bacterium and is not affected by antibiotics, it needs no prompting to colonize the vagina, which it finds devoid of its natural bacterial competitors. Once the fungus has dug itself into the vagina, it is difficult to dislodge and the normal bacteria, particularly the lactobacillus, find it hard to re-establish themselves.

In pregnancy a change in the hormonal balance has an effect on the vagina and, again, *Candida albicans* finds conditions more favourable. The oral contraceptive pill, particularly if containing much oestrogen, has an effect on the vagina similar to pregnancy. Vulvo-vaginal candidal infection is not only more common among pill-takers and pregnant women, but is also rather more difficult to eradicate.

Other factors encouraging the development of candidal infection, or making it more difficult to cope with, are treatment with drugs containing corticosteroids or those which depress the body's natural immunity. Candidal infection is more common among diabetics, where the excess sugar in the urine seems to encourage the growth of the fungus.

One of the features of *Candida albicans* that makes it such a tiresome organism is its ability to 'sensitize' individuals. Rather in the same way that the mite of scabies sets up an allergic reaction, in certain people infected with candida an intense irritation occurs, which may be quite out of proportion to the degree of infection.

Symptoms and signs in women. In both men and women the signs and symptoms of candidal infection can be divided into those caused by the infection itself and those caused by the 'allergic' reaction to the fungus. When the vagina is heavily colonized by *C. albicans* there is a noticeable change in the vaginal discharge. The discharge may be thicker than usual, indeed it is sometimes described by the patient as being 'curd-like'. This appearance like cottage cheese is not that common; more often a thinner white discharge is complained of. There are not usually other 'internal' symptoms, because the vagina is poorly supplied by sensory nerve endings and itching *inside* the vagina is not common. The same is not true for the vaginal entrance and vulva. There may be the most intense pruritus all over the external genitalia and blood may be drawn as a result of the vigorous scratching this induces. The skin may take on a white, waxy appearance with thin slits or 'cuts' on the surface. The skin between the vagina and the anus is commonly involved, and the anus itself may be raw and red as a result of the intense irritation.

Occasionally, the infection may spread to involve the natal cleft, the fold between the buttocks, behind the anus.

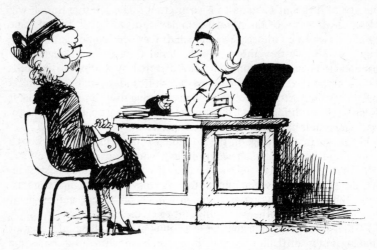

'Why didn't you tell me about this before, Mother?'

The symptoms and signs described above are those seen in someone who is sensitized to the fungus. It is surprising to find some women who are heavily infected with candida and yet who deny any symptoms save an increase in vaginal discharge. They are, however, the exception rather than the rule.

Candidal infection in men. Candidal infection of the penis is much less common than infection of the female genitalia. There are sound anatomical reasons for this — the distance of the penis from the anus militates against direct infection from that source, and the 'external' nature of the penis makes it more easy to keep clean and perhaps abort an early infection. If actual infection is uncommon, a balanitis due to *C. albicans* is not; but this is more often due to the 'allergic' type of response to infection in the sexual partner. Some males are able to diagnose vaginal thrush in their wives or girl-friends within seconds of the start of sexual intercourse because of the immediate reaction that is set up. It is the uncircumcised male who is most likely to acquire an actual *infection* with *C. albicans*, but, like the female, he does not have to develop symptoms. Occasionally the fungus can ensconce itself in the terminal portion of the urethra, and it may then give rise to symptoms similar to those found in non-specific urethritis.

Candidal infection may be passed between practising male homosexuals with similar penile or anal soreness and itching.

Treatment. There has grown up a folk belief that recurrent thrush is completely untreatable. This stems from the fact that candidal infection does often recur, and one of the reasons for these recurrences is inadequate treatment. It is axiomatic that all the sites that are infected should be treated if there is to be any hope of cure. This means that the vagina, vulva, and perineal and perianal skin, as well as the intestine, should have antifungal treatment. Unlike many antibiotics, the antifungal agents commonly used are not absorbed from the gut and it is therefore not effective just to give tablets or capsules by mouth. These will certainly be needed to clear the bowel of candida, but it is also necessary to treat the vagina with fungicidal pessaries, and the intervening skin with cream or ointment if there is to be any chance of success.

In some people cure will be achieved more easily than in others. There may be one or more unfavourable factors at work in the resistant case. The taking of broad-spectrum antibiotics, pregnancy, and the oral contraceptive are the commonest causes of difficulty; however the first two are not, or should not be, permanent, and it should be possible to eliminate thrush even if the pill is continued, by giving a prolonged course of treatment.

To what extent is vaginal candidiasis a sexually transmitted disease? Probably rather less than immediately appears, for, although symptoms of thrush may seem to be related to a recent sexual act, it may be that the trauma of vigorous sexual intercourse has brought to the surface that which was lying dormant. That is not to say that sexual partners of people with recurrent candidal infection should not be sought and examined – many cases of treatment-resistant thrush are due to repeated reinfection by an asymptomatic carrier. If there is a likelihood of reinfection, use of the fungicidal cream as a lubricant during intercourse or intercourse after insertion of a fungicidal pessary are relatively painless methods of treating the male sexual partner.

Trichomonas vaginalis

This organism is the second most common identifiable cause of vaginal discharge, and if candida produces the itchiest, trichomonas produces the most evil-smelling. *Trichomonas vaginalis* is a protozoon, a one-celled animal which moves about by means of flagellae which work like flexible oars from the broad end of this pear-shaped organism. Protozoa are much larger than bacteria or viruses, although still not visible to the naked eye. Other species of animal are affected by these sorts of organism – horses suffer from a sexually transmitted disease due to *Trichomonas equus*.

It has been calculated that, at some point in her life, one woman in five will be infected with this parasite and it is also generally accepted that the organism is almost exclusively sexually transmitted. Those who postulate a non-sexual mode of transmission refer to documented infection in pre-pubertal virgins, the low rate of isolation in males, the occasional finding of the organism in swimming pools and spa waters, and the fact that infection could be acquired from lavatories. Evidence for this latter theory followed an unusual and ingenious bit of medical research. Following the use of a lavatory by a woman with vaginal trichomoniasis, the medical team dropped small blocks of wood of the same size and shape as faeces into the pan and caught the resultant splashes on culture plates. It was possible to grow *Trichomonas vaginalis* from these plates. There have also been well annotated studies of the transmission of trichomonal infection to the newborn offspring of mothers harbouring the organism, but not to the children of uninfected mothers. Although these various studies have demonstrated that TV *can* be acquired other than sexually, as with gonorrhoea, such cases probably make up a very small minority of the total.

Although some women with trichomonal infection in the vagina may remain symptomless, the majority will develop at least a vaginal discharge. This is typically a thin, irritant discharge with a characteristic 'fishy' odour, and any skin that comes into contact with it tends to become excoriated and sore. There develops as a result both a vaginitis and a vulvitis which make intercourse, if not impossible, extremely uncomfortable. There may also be some bleeding after intercourse. Dysuria may occur as a result of the urine coming into contact with inflamed skin. This sometimes leads to the mistaken treatment of trichomonal infection as cystitis.

In many cases trichomonal infection is associated with other diseases, and while few would advocate the routine screening for other infection of all women found to be suffering from candidal infection, the finding of *Trichomonas vaginalis* is an absolute indication for further investigation to exclude other sexually transmitted disease. Between 30 and 50 per cent of women with gonorrhoea have coincidental trichomoniasis and up to 40 per cent of women with TV have gonorrhoea — the figures vary between different centres and depend on the group of women being examined.

In the male, *Trichomonas vaginalis* usually affects the urethra and the symptoms that it produces are less than those found with gonococcal or other non-gonococcal causes of urethritis. The discharge is usually a thin mucoid or white one and it may, like the vaginal discharge in women, be frothy. There will be some dysuria as well, if the discharge is heavy. It seems that many men, however, show little in the way of symptoms and may therefore pass on the disease quite unknowingly. The infection can involve the prostate gland and the seminal vesicles and this may produce urgency of micturition or haematospermia (the finding of blood in the ejaculate). While the woman has no natural way of eliminating the infection, it is probable that many men carry the infection in the urethra for a matter of a few days only, after which the flushing action of passing urine may eliminate the organisms.

Perhaps because of this washing effect of urination, attempts to identify the infection in male contacts of women with TV are very often unsuccessful. As a rule only about 10 per cent of such men can be shown to have the organism when only urethral tests are taken. If fluid from the prostate and a specimen of the ejaculate are also examined, however, the diagnosis rate increases markedly, and over 70 per cent of male contacts were shown to be harbouring the organism in one series where these exhaustive tests were carried out.

In women it is probably the easiest infection to diagnose. A simple microscopic examination of some vaginal discharge, suspended in a salt solution, will give the diagnosis in most cases, and there are also reliable methods of culturing it in the laboratory. It is seen quite easily on the specially stained smear tests (Papanicolaou smear) for cancer of the cervix. This is just as well because trichomonal infection causes changes in the cells of the cervix which mimic those that precede cancerous changes. Such changes, when caused by trichomonal infection, are rapidly reversible with anti-protozoal treatment.

There is a strange, as yet unexplained, difference between ethnic groups in their incidence of trichomonal infection. It is found significantly more often in the coloured races, both male and female, and whether this is due to some actual racial difference in susceptibility, or whether it simply reflects some general difference in the social pattern of spread of the disease is not clear.

There are several drugs available which are highly effective at eliminating trichomonas from both sexes, and metronidazole is both the earliest and most widely used of these. Courses of treatment vary from one to seven days and although it is always preferable to examine the male sexual partner of an infected woman, because of the difficulties of making the diagnosis in men it is sometimes justifiable to treat the male without confirming the diagnosis, particularly if it can be shown that reinfection has taken place.

Haemophilus vaginalis. This rod-shaped bacterium is a not uncommon cause of an offensive vaginal discharge in women. There is debate as to the extent to which it is sexually transmitted, but in some reports up to 70 per cent of male partners of infected women have been shown to harbour the organism. It is probable that, in the majority of male cases, haemophilus does not produce a urethritis and most men with the infection will have neither signs nor symptoms.

Some women who are infected with this bacterium have little in the way of symptoms, but the majority will have noticed an increase in their vaginal discharge. There may be a vulvo-vaginitis and the discharge is sometimes frothy like that found in trichomonal infection. Although this organism does respond to treatment with certain antibiotics, it is, surprisingly, more sensitive to metronidazole, the anti-protozoal agent used to treat trichomonas.

Group-B streptococci. This ubiquitous group of gram-positive cocci are particularly prevalent among women attending special clinics. Although they are probably sexually transmitted, they do not appear to produce much in the way of symptoms in either men or women. In particular, they are not associated with non-gonococcal urethritis and do not produce a typical vaginal discharge. Their importance, like that of cytomegalovirus, lies in their propensity for causing serious perinatal infection. They are capable of causing meningitis, septicaemia, and severe pneumonia in the newborn, complications that are, thankfully, rare.

Foreign bodies

A small proportion of vaginal discharges are due to foreign bodies. As with males, this is not a reference to the side-effects of hot-blooded Latin lovers, but means any object that is found in the body but is not of the body. The intra-uterine device is a foreign body, as are the tampons used to absorb the menstrual flow. The latter are sometimes forgotten and left in the vagina at the end of a period and may be responsible for a persistent, foul, vaginal discharge, which is, however, easy to treat.

While children are notoriously prone to insert small objects into their ears or noses, the dawn of adult sexual awakening heralds a second phase of insertion in both males and females, at first in an exploratory fashion and then as an adjunct to masturbation or to heighten sexual pleasure. Hence the succession of men and women who arrive in casualty departments with vibrators irretrievably lost in the rectum.

Case history. Miss Bridget T., as a fourteen-year-old schoolgirl, inserted a hairpin into her vagina and was unable to retrieve it. She was too frightened and embarrassed to tell her parents about the missing object, and since she didn't develop any untoward effects she dismissed the problem from her mind. When she was nineteen she had been going out with a steady boyfriend for three years, and they had decided to get married. She went to her GP to ask him to prescribe the oral contraceptive and, before he prescribed the pill, he examined her thoroughly, including a vaginal examination. He was considerably taken aback when he felt two sharp prongs projecting down into the vagina beside the cervix. During the preceding years the hairpin had perforated the inner end of the vagina and eventually turned through $180°$. It took a minor

PLATE 3

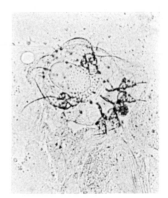

The mite of scabies

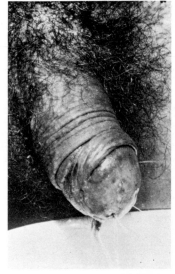

Late gonorrhoea: multiple
urethral fistulae*

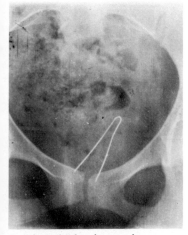

Foreign body in vagina: see
Chapter 6

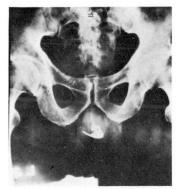

Foreign body in urethra: see
Chapter 5*

*Reproduced with permission from King & Nicol (1975) Venereal Diseases,
(3rd edn, Ballière Tindall, London).

PLATE 4

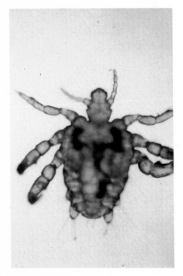

'Crab' louse

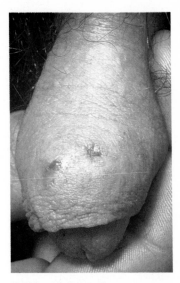

Scabies of the penis

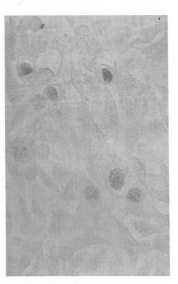

Chlamydia trachomatis in cell culture

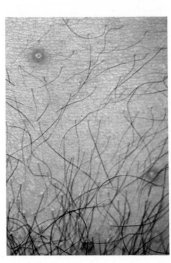

Molluscum contagiosum in pubic area

surgical operation to remove the pin and Miss T. suffered no ill-effects and was able to start her sexual life without inflicting grievous injury on her unsuspecting fiancé.

Honeymoon cystitis and the urethral syndrome

Honeymoon cystitis, with its descriptive and emotive label, is badly named, because it by no means restricts itself to married couples on honeymoon, whatever small proportion of such couples, these days, wait until their honeymoon for their first sexual experience together. It describes a syndrome, sometimes related to the first intercourse but by no means restricted to it, in which the woman develops the symptoms of cystitis, particularly frequency and dysuria, following sex. There may be some local discomfort following the first ever sexual intercourse related to the tearing of the hymen, but honeymoon cystitis as often crops up in women who are sexually experienced for whom other explanations must be sought. Obviously the symptoms may actually be due to an infection of the bladder — such infections are certainly more common among women who are sexually active than among those who are not — and the symptoms may be due, if not to a sexually transmitted disease, to other minor infections such as thrush; but in many cases no bacteriological offender is found to account for the symptoms.

Perhaps the most common cause is simple mechanical trauma, and allied to this, poor vulval and vaginal lubrication. Lubrication in the woman, like erection in the man, is not under conscious control and cannot be turned on or off at will. If the woman is nervous, apprehensive, or frightened, or if sexual foreplay has been either inadequate or incompetent, then she is likely, quite literally, to dry up. This may well make the act of intercourse uncomfortable and batter and bruise the external genitalia and the opening of the urethra. Following this there may be discomfort on urination, and a vicious circle is started in which memory of previous discomfort combines with apprehension at the possibility of its recurring and perpetuates the nervousness or fear that was responsible in the first place.

It is important to exclude the more obvious infective causes by a thorough microbiological examination and, once this has been done, advice on the use of artificial lubricants is enough to break the vicious circle in many cases. If the lubricant can be applied by the man during sexual foreplay, there will be an improvement in the sex act and the troublesome urinary symptoms will disappear as well. The other piece of useful advice is that the woman should pass water as soon as possible after intercourse, as this too seems to make this recurrent problem less likely.

The urethral syndrome is really outside the scope of this book, indeed whole books themselves have been devoted to it. The syndrome would be regarded by many as including honeymoon cystitis, that is to say urethral symptoms related to sexual intercourse, but also covers a host of other bacteria-negative causes. It is probably a mistake to regard the urethral syndrome as one single condition rather as it would be wrong to think of 'pneumonia' as being a single disease of the lungs. Some patients landed with this label will have viral cystitis, difficult to diagnose by the the standard methods of analysing the urine, others will have one of the genital infections like trichomoniasis, candida, or herpes while some actually have a bacterial infection of the bladder or kidney that has been missed. However, even after excluding these infective causes and any anatomical reasons (it has been suggested, for instance, that a 'pouting' urethral meatus in women can give rise to recurrent urethral symptoms, and a urethral caruncle, a tiny button of sensitive flesh at the urethral opening, can certainly cause a similar discomfort), there remain a few women for whom no predisposing factor can be elicited. What can be said is that those whose discomfort is related to intercourse are most likely to be cured of their symptoms either by a combination of improved lubrication and post-coital urination, or by treating any infection that underlies the symptoms.

7

Virus infections

It is not surprising that some viruses have taken advantage of the sexual act as a vehicle for their transmission, but, while bacteria such as gonococci, treponemes, and the organisms responsible for the tropical sexually transmitted diseases have become so specialized that non-venereal transmission is extremely rare, the sexually transmitted virus infections, with the exception of genital warts, are frequently transmitted in other ways as well.

While many viruses *can* be transmitted sexually, there are five conditions whose spread is commonly by sexual contact. They are: Herpes genitalis, molluscum contagiosum, condylomata acuminata, Australia antigen-positive hepatitis, and cytomegalovirus infection.

Herpes simplex

The virus of herpes simplex is probably the most common human viral parasite after that responsible for the common cold. It causes sores on the lips, face, eyes, and mouth, on the genitalia, occasionally elsewhere on the skin, and rarely causes a very serious infection in the central nervous system of the newborn. There appear to be two distinct types of herpes simplex virus – type I (herpes labialis or facialis) which is found predominantly above the neck and type II (herpes genitalis) more often found in the genital and anal areas. Over 60 per cent of children aged five can be shown to have been infected with herpes virus, and this figure approaches 95 per cent in adults. Once infected, people remain carriers of the virus for life, some of them suffering repeated attacks while others build up enough resistance to remain free of symptoms. The most usual mode of transmission of type I herpes is kissing, and following exposure a susceptible individual will develop a crop of blisters (vesicles) on the lips after about four days. These are itchy and painful and eventually crust over before disappearing after a further week or two. Alternatively, the infection may be confined to the inside of the mouth, where it may not produce any symptoms, or may cause ulceration which is difficult to distinguish from 'aphthous' ulcers (the small mouth ulcers that are so common and so difficult to treat). Infection is therefore not necessarily associated with any symptoms and the majority of type I infections probably go undiagnosed and unrecognized.

At the time of the first attack it is possible to measure an increase in antibody levels in the blood, but these seem to remain fairly steady in any further attacks. There is, then, a vast reservoir of herpes infection in the community, much of which is undiagnosed. The virus lies dormant in the tissues and will manifest itself, in those who suffer symptomatic recurrences, following a variety of provocatory factors. These include trauma, sunlight, high fever, and general debility. With time these 'cold sores' become less frequent and the severity of the attacks diminishes.

Herpes genitalis. Herpes virus is the commonest cause of genital ulceration in the United Kingdom, and, in those who suffer repeated recurrences, is one of the most harrowing of the sexually transmitted diseases. Although infection with type II virus is the rule and is usually acquired through contact with the sexual partner's infected genitalia, type I infection following mouth-to-genital contact is becoming increasingly common. The virus is highly infectious to those who have not previously been exposed to it, but the majority of people have a degree of immunity due to past clinical or symptomless mouth or face infection. Indeed it is unusual to find a fresh case of genital herpes in someone who has a history of cold sores, although it does occur in some cases.

In the susceptible man who is exposed to infection, the first signs develop after four or five days. The earliest symptom is a slight itching in the genital area, which within twenty-four hours gives way to discrete irritating vesicles one or two millimetres in diameter. These little blisters enlarge and eventually burst to form ulcers which are shallow and acutely painful to touch. In this primary attack, there may be marked constitutional upset with fever and flu-like illness. Secondary bacterial infection of the ulcers is common and there is a marked swelling of the lymph nodes in the groin, which can be very tender. The diagnosis may be made with a high degree of accuracy from the clinical appearance of the lesions, and this can be comfirmed by growing the virus in the laboratory on developing hens' eggs.

Although the shaft of the penis is the site most often affected, the glans penis and the coronal sulcus are sometimes infected and, rarely, the infection may start inside the urethra. In such cases, the symptoms are those of an acute urethritis with a mucoid or muco-purulent discharge. If this is not diagnosed and recurrences occur at the same site, the patient will be labelled as a refractory case of non-specific urethritis and may be subjected to prolonged courses of antibiotic treatment, which, of course, will have no effect on the course of the disease.

Following the primary attack, there may be no further episodes, or the disease may recur over a long period, in some cases several years. No recurrent attack is ever as bad as the primary one, and the frequency, severity, and duration of subsequent attacks all tend to diminish. As with herpes of the lip there are certain provoking factors which tend to precipitate an attack. Unfortunately, one of these is sexual intercourse, where the trauma of the sex act rather than reinfection causes the recurrence.

A first attack of herpes in the adult, sexually active woman can often go undiagnosed because the primary lesions may be hidden away in the folds of the labia and close examination is needed to identify the ulceration. The vesicles are often found on the labia or around the vaginal entrance. Sometimes they may spread to involve the anus and perianal skin. In a proportion of cases the first site of infection is the cervix, when there may not be any local pain. Sometimes there is a double infection of the cervix and the external genitalia. There may be marked swelling and considerable pain in the genital region, and there are usually enlarged glands in the groin which are very tender to the touch.

One of the reasons for difficulty in diagnosing this condition when it first occurs is the apparent similarity of the symptoms that it produces to those associated with cystitis. The herpetic lesions may involve the opening of the urethra and in some cases the infection spreads to the bladder. Whether this happens or not, one of the main symptoms is dysuria — pain on passing urine. If this symptom is analysed closely, it will be found that it is 'external' in character. That is, the pain is caused by urine running over the acutely painful ulcers. This is in contrast to the dysuria associated with cystitis where the discomfort is actually *urethral*. There may be frequency of micturition and, in a proportion of cases, these symptoms may progress to acute retention of urine, when the hapless female finds it impossible to pass urine at all. Women, like men, may suffer moderate systemic upset, and any secondary bacterial infection may need to be treated with antibiotics.

First attacks may last longer in women than in men. Recurrent attacks are common and may follow on as soon as one week after the end of the primary attack. Again there are several precipitating factors which may lead to repeated recurrence, with sexual intercourse heading the list, but the attacks will tend to become less frequent and severe.

Case history. Pamela T., a 28-year-old airline stewardess, had attended a department of genito-urinary medicine for three years with recurrent herpes genitalis. She had a steady boyfriend who had never suffered from herpes himself, and, after a difficult first year following her primary attack, she had gradually improved until she finally went nine months without any trouble. She arrived one day in the clinic in the peak of health and triumphantly announced that she had just got married and was setting out to live in Palm Springs with her husband. Some six months later an anguished letter arrived from the United States in which she said that since arriving in the USA she had barely had two weeks without an attack of herpes and could she possibly attend again when she was next in England. When she was seen there seemed to be no good reason for this strange reversal in her clinical course. Her husband didn't suffer from herpes, there had been no increase in the frequency of sexual intercourse, and there had been no inter-current infection to explain the setback. When she was examined, she did indeed have a nasty attack of herpes, but the doctor who looked at her noticed that she was as brown as a berry. All over. It transpired that there was a secluded roof on her house where she was wont to sunbathe totally naked. It was gently suggested to her that in future, for reasons other than decency, she should wear a pair of bikini pants when sunbathing. She followed this advice and had no further attacks of herpes in the next six months. Ultraviolet light has long been accepted as a provocative factor for herpes of the face and lips and many people find that their annual attack coincides with their visit to Majorca or trip to the ski slopes.

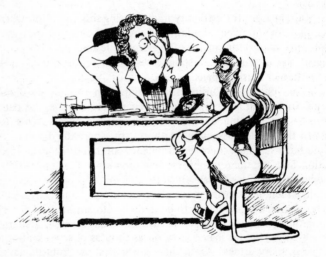

'When I said a virus could be airborne, I wasn't really thinking of the back seat of a D.C. 10.

If herpetic infection is confined to the cervix, the only symptom is likely to be an excess of muco-purulent vaginal discharge. There may also be a degree of enlargement of the lymph nodes in the groin.

There is no satisfactory treatment for herpes simplex infections and the best that can be offered is medication to ease the symptoms and possibly cut short an attack, and advice on how to cope with the problems that recurrent herpes brings. Antibiotics have no effect on viruses, and the only indication for their use in herpetic infection is the presence of superadded, or secondary infection by bacteria. There are several 'anti-viral' products available but their topical application, recommended by several authorities, has yet to be shown to have any convincing therapeutic effect. Idoxuridine, one such agent, can be applied to herpetic ulcers either in an ointment base or dissolved in a solvent which aids its absorption in the skin, and has enthusiastic followers, but again convincing evidence of its efficacy is lacking. This drug has been used to good effect in generalized viral infections, when it can be injected directly into the blood-stream, but this is not without hazard and is not indicated unless the infection is life-threatening.

Application of ether or certain vital dyes to the ulcers both have their adherents but seem to have little effect on the natural course of the disease. Creams and ointments containing corticosteroids, because of their powerful anti-inflammatory action, can lessen the symptoms considerably but they also have the effect of damping down the body's natural defences and, in theory, could lead to the spread of the infection, with potentially fatal results in a primary attack when there is no natural immunity at all. Smallpox vaccination has its advocates, on the principle that it may stimulate the body's immune responses generally, but, again, there is no good evidence for its efficacy. Recently a new group of drugs, cytosine and adenosine arabinoside, have been used with considerable success against generalized viral illness, particularly in people whose natural defence mechanisms are below par, but it remains to be seen whether it is feasible to use them on localized herpetic infection.

In the last few years there has been a succession of reports, mostly emanating from the continent of Europe, claiming good results from vaccines against herpes virus. With no exceptions these results have been based on poorly controlled trials which, although they do not show that herpes vaccines *don't* work, certainly do not prove that they do. More important than any lack of efficacy is the very real risk that vaccines prepared from killed or attenuated virus particles may contain carcinogenic elements. It has been shown that inactivated herpes virus is more capable of inducing cancerous change in certain cells than the normal virus, and the possible risks attached to such vaccines vastly outweigh any dubious advantages. In the United States work is being done on a vaccine which consists only of the outer covering of the virus particle and so avoids the dangers of using the virus's nucleic acid core. So far it has been used only in animal experiments, but it certainly seems effective in reducing the severity of attacks of herpes in guinea-pigs.

The treatment of acute retention of urine occurring in a primary herpetic attack in the female deserves a brief mention. Such cases will often have been treated as acute cystitis for a day or two, and may present to the casualty department or emergency room with a bladder so swollen that it mimics a twenty week pregnancy. As already stated, the reason for the retention is the exquisite pain associated with passing urine, and the best way of solving the problem is to apply some local anaesthetic ointment until the vulva and external genitalia are completely numb and then sit the patient in a warm bath until urine has been passed. Occasionally it may be necessary to pass a urinary catheter to drain the bladder, but this is avoided, if possible, for the procedure may itself introduce infection.

People with recurrent herpes soon get to know their disease well and can often tell 24 hours before the vesicles appear that an attack is imminent. They are advised that they are potentially highly infectious when the ulcers are present and should refrain from intercourse (should they feel like it) until the attack has passed off. Probably less than 50 per cent of patients who develop genital herpes go on to have recurrent attacks, and in only a small proportion of these do the attacks occur so frequently as to disrupt life appreciably.

Very rarely, a newborn infant contracts herpes simplex and goes on to develop an acute viral infection of the brain, which is almost invariably fatal. In these cases the infection has been contracted during passage through the birth canal from sores on the mother's genitalia. This only occurs if the mother has developed a *primary* attack in the last few weeks of pregnancy. She will have no natural antibodies to the infection and therefore will not have passed any such antibodies to her baby via the placenta. If the mother develops a *recurrent* attack just before giving birth, her antibodies will protect the child from this severe infection. When a primary attack occurs in such circumstances, there is a strong case for delivering the baby by caesarian section.

Carcinoma of the cervix. This cancer, which, after cancer of the breast, is the most common neoplasm in women, has many features in common with the sexually transmitted diseases. The same groups of women are at risk: those of a promiscuous nature, and particularly those whose first sexual intercourse occurred at an early age. It is virtually never seen in celibate women and one very large survey in the United States failed to detect a single case among 30 000 nuns. Another study which looked at men whose wives had died of cancer of the cervix has shown that there is a much higher incidence of cervical cancer among their *second wives* than would be expected by chance. Because viruses are known to be implicated in the development of certain cancers, it was natural to investigate any possible relationship between herpes infection of the cervix and cervical cancer. Although there is no certain association between the two, the fact that both occur in a similar group of women suggests that some care should be taken in following up women who have suffered from herpetic infection of the cervix. Instead of the more normal five-yearly cervical smear tests that are recommended for all adult females, it may be wiser to repeat this test every two years instead.

Molluscum contagiosum

This skin condition, caused by a large 'pox' virus, has been thought over the years to be restricted to children living in crowded, closed communities and adults who attend Turkish baths or indulge in all-in wrestling. It is now clear, however, that its most important mode of transmission is a sexual one. In itself it is of no great importance, but it may serve as a pointer to the presence of other sexually transmitted infection. Over 80 per cent of cases in one series were either suffering from or had suffered from other sexually transmitted diseases.

The lesions consist of separate, raised, umbilicated spots which vary from one millimetre to one centimetre in diameter. They are orangey-pink in colour with a pearly, opalescent top. They contain, rather like a blackhead, a plug of material which can be expressed if the lesion is squeezed.

They are found on the external genitalia and on the thighs, buttocks, and lower abdomen. Up to 80 may be found, although there are usually less than 10. The incubation period may be up to three months and, like warts, they may appear in crops. They are treated by curetting or by digging a sharpened orange stick dipped in acid or phenol into the centre of the lesion.

Hepatitis

Hepatitis simply means an inflammatory disorder of the liver and it can be caused by a variety of agents: drugs and poisons, bacteria and viruses. Viral hepatitis has been recognized since the Second World War as being divisible into two distinct types. These were described as *infectious* or type A hepatitis, where the method of transmission was faecal/oral, and *serum* or type B hepatitis, in which contact with blood or blood-products from an infected person was necessary. The incubation period for type A hepatitis was accepted as being much shorter than those for serum hepatitis, but research into either form of hepatitis was hampered by an inability to identify the causative agent. A major breakthrough came in the middle sixties when an antigen was isolated from an Aborigine who was suffering from hepatitis. In contrast to the majority of medical discoveries which are jealously named after their progenitor, the Aborigine was anonymously honoured by calling the agent 'Australia antigen'.

It is now fairly certain that the Australia antigen represents part of the virus responsible for type B hepatitis and its discovery has made it easier to determine the modes of transmission and the presence of a 'carrier' state, in which the infected person may suffer no ill health from his disease but is still capable of passing it on to others.

Armed with this tool for diagnosing asymptomatic carriers of the infection and those who had been infected in the past, several screening studies were undertaken in the early seventies, and to many people's surprise the incidence of past and present infection was found to be very high amongst those attending departments of venereology or genito-urinary medicine. When the results were further analysed, it was shown that this high incidence was largely due to the male homosexual population attending these clinics. Later work has convincingly demonstrated that sexual contact is an important, if not the most important, method of spread of hepatitis-associated antigen in urban communities.

The method of spread is not clear, but may be related to the more traumatic effects of anal intercourse when abrasions and tears of the skin can occur. A high percentage of the homosexuals who are found to be positive, practise fellatio and, in particular, allowed ejaculation to take place in the mouth and then swallowed the semen. Analyses of semen have demonstrated the presence of antigen, but failed to show levels as high as those in the blood. What is not in dispute is that the male homosexual, as with syphilis, is at great risk of catching this infection.

Probably, the majority of people infected with the virus of type B hepatitis will suffer no important consequences. Some will have clinical illness with jaundice. The majority of these will get over this, although remaining a risk to those people with whom they come into contact. Others, however, will develop a chronic and progressive malfunction of the liver that may lead to total liver failure. There is some evidence that the sexually transmitted form of hepatitis is more likely to lead to liver damage than that passed on by means of blood products. It should be a standard procedure for all clinics dealing with the sexually transmitted diseases to screen their homosexual patients for Australia antigen.

Genital warts

These warts, also known as condylomata acuminata, are, like common skin warts, caused by a virus. They are almost exclusively sexually transmitted and are very rarely found other than in the ano-genital region. Plain skin warts are also found on the genitals and in such cases a sexual mode of transmission need not be postulated.

If the virus from genital warts is examined with the electron microscope it is not morphologically distinguishable from that causing skin warts, but there may be some minor antigenic differences between the two types. There appears to be a much higher concentration of virus particles in the lesions of genital as opposed to skin warts.

Certainly, the appearance of the two sorts of warts is very different, skin warts being usually less than 5 mm in diameter and flattish, while the genital variety are more pointed and 'frond-like', and may grow to considerable size. The only site other than the ano-genital region where they may be found is in the mouth and, when there, they have usually been acquired sexually. The incubation period may be up to one year, and this makes it difficult in many cases to decide from whom the warts have been caught; not only that, but they often seem to have been seeded on the principle adhered to by market gardeners, to give successive crops over a long period. No sooner has one lot been dealt with, than another appears to take its place.

Warts are slightly more common in uncircumcised males. They can be found on the shaft of the penis and on the glans, but their predilection for a damp and warm environment makes them most often seen under the foreskin. Sometimes they may spread to involve the terminal urethra, and can only be seen if the urethral meatus is parted. They may then be an unusual cause of non-specific urethritis. They do not produce many symptoms. Occasional itching may occur, but more usually it is the appearance of these growths on the penis which prompts the sufferer to seek treatment. Male homosexuals frequently have warts around the anal margin and in some cases these extend up into the anal canal itself. Anal warts are seven times more common than penile warts among homosexuals.

In women, warts tend to go unnoticed unless they are quite large. They are therefore diagnosed, as often as not, as a chance finding during examination. They can be found anywhere on the external genitalia, on the vaginal walls, and on the cervix. They seem to flourish where there is a lot of moisture, and it is quite common to find a coincidental vaginal infection with a marked discharge. It is difficult to eradicate the warts until the discharge has been treated. For reasons as yet unexplained, genital warts proliferate markedly during pregnancy, and they can assume gigantic proportions if left untreated. They do, however, tend to regress rapidly after childbirth. Perianal warts are frequently found at the same time as genital warts and there need be no assumption that anal intercourse has taken place, although it will have done so in some 50 per cent of cases. Warts have more nuisance value than medical significance, but, like all of the minor sexually transmitted diseases, they serve as a useful indicator to the possibility of other infection, and anyone with anal or genital warts should make sure that they are screened for other genital infections.

'In the male, if a prepuce is present, circumcision is carried out.' So reads a textbook on the venereal diseases published in 1940. Nowadays, most physicians would regard this as an over-radical approach to the problem of warts but it does reflect the despair, by no means restricted to those days, felt by doctors trying to cope with recurrent genital condylomata. Although it is possible to detect antibodies to wart virus in the blood of infected individuals, these antibodies, rather like those found in cases of syphilis, reflect the body's recognition of the infection rather than any intention, let alone ability, to dispose of it. It is certainly true that in many cases warts will regress and even disappear without any treatment, but it is unclear why this should happen and there is no way of predicting which sufferers will be able to rid themselves of the warts or how to stimulate the body's defences to that end.

In both men and women the first line of treatment is the application of substances to the warts. These may be caustic, such as trichloroacetic acid or phenol, or anti-mitotic (acting on the virus-infected cell to stop it dividing), like podophylline, which is an extract of a fungus. If the warts are very extensive or if local applications have failed, then the warts can be frozen, using liquid nitrogen, or burnt off with electro-cautery. All these treatments have variable and unpredictable success because of the 'cropping' nature of the warts, and the ever-present possibility of reinfection by the sexual partner. Sometimes they won't go away because of plain orneryness. With both sexes it is important to examine the sexual partners, 60 per cent of whom will be found to have genital warts. In the female it is important to treat any cause of vaginal discharge.

Cytomegalovirus

Cytomagalovirus (CMV) is a virus with many similarities to the herpes virus. In the adult, infection may lead to a disease similar to glandular fever with enlargement of the liver and spleen, a rash, and, in more severe cases, pneumonia. The afflicted person will complain of aches and pains, headache, sore throat, loss of appetite, and general malaise. The main importance of the virus, however, lies in its capacity to infect the foetus *in utero*. If the infection is passed on by the mother, the baby has a 75 per cent chance of having some neurological disorder, ranging from deafness and blindness to spastic paralysis. It is an infection, like herpes, of world-wide distribution, and 50 per cent of women of childbearing age show evidence of antibodies to CMV in their blood. When there is active infection, the virus can be found in saliva, urine, vaginal discharge, and semen.

It can certainly be passed on by kissing, and there has recently been strong epidemiological evidence that CMV infection can be sexually transmitted.

It should perhaps, like type B hepatitis, be added to the list of diseases that are often or even *usually* passed on in this way. After

Virus infections

symptoms of infection have disappeared, the virus may stay around the body for some considerable time, and it is often possible to grow it as long as one year after the infection has taken place.

8

Syphilis

Syphilis has a reputation in the United Kingdom today quite out of proportion to the amount of infection that it causes. Like the 'bogeyman' used by mother to frighten her recalcitrant children into better behaviour, syphilis or 'the pox' is used by scaremongering educators to put the fear of God into those people they think might be at risk of catching VD. It is a very rare disease today and the incidence has decreased markedly since the Second World War. Having followed the decline in the number of cases of gonorrhoea into the middle fifties, syphilis, in contrast, has remained at a comparatively low level ever since. There has, however, been a change in the ratio of men to women with the disease. This is a reflection of the fact that practising male homosexuals are particularly at risk of catching syphilis, while the incidence among male and female heterosexuals continues to decrease.

Syphilis is caused by an unusual micro-organism called *Treponema pallidum*, a thin, spiral, flexible bacterium which moves with a combination of corkscrew and bending movements. It has proved impossible to grow the treponeme in the laboratory on normal growth media, and this has hampered research into the organism. At the present time it can be inoculated into laboratory animals, in which it will multiply, and will produce an illness similar to the human disease in the higher apes.

Syphilis is seen in two main forms – acquired and congenital. The acquired form of the disease is almost invariably the result of sexual activity with an infected person, while congenital syphilis, as its name implies, is passed on passively while the developing foetus is *in utero*.

Early syphilis

It is generally accepted that the treponeme needs a small cut or abrasion in the skin before it can gain entry and cause an infection; simple contact with the skin is not enough. This has been postulated as one of the reasons for the disease being more common among male homosexuals – anal intercourse being more traumatic than vaginal intercourse and being more likely to cause skin tears. The incubation period for primary syphilis is between one and twelve weeks, with the majority of cases showing evidence of infection at two to four weeks. The incubation period almost certainly varies with the number of bacteria originally passed on. The treponeme, once in the tissues, multiplies locally and also travels to the nearby lymph nodes, where further division and multiplication takes place. As a result of the infection, the small blood-vessels supplying the skin become blocked and the resulting diminution of the blood-supply leads to local death of tissue, which manifests itself as the primary chancre.

This primary sore is usually a solitary ulcer, and by the time it has appeared the local lymph nodes are invariably involved and treatment of the chancre with antiseptics or antibiotic ointments will have no effect on progression of the disease. In men the commonest site of infection is the penis. The ulcer is usually found on the glans penis or the foreskin, although it is sometimes found at the base of the shaft of the penis – the so-called 'condom chancre'. In such cases the unlucky individual has taken the precaution of wearing a contraceptive sheath, but a sore on the vulva, say, of his sexual partner has come into contact with part of the penis not covered by the condom.

In women the lesion of primary syphilis will be found on the labia majora or minora, on the clitoris, or around the urethral meatus. A chancre is also sometimes found on the cervix and rarely on the vaginal wall. Although there may be quite considerable local swelling, in many cases the lesion will go unnoticed. The ulcer in both sexes has a hard floor, which may feel like a small button just under the skin surface, varying in size from the barely discernible to the size of a finger-nail. Although it has a malevolent appearance, the primary chancre is usually completely painless and, unless secondary bacterial infection occurs, there may be no symptoms. Like the female, the male homosexual may have a symptomless ulcer. Although the genitalia are the most likely sites for a chancre to be found, they also occur around the anus in both sexes and are occasionally seen on the lips, tongue, or nipple.

The sore of primary syphilis is followed after six to eight weeks by the development of the secondary stage. The primary sore may still be present in about one third of cases of secondary syphilis.

In secondary syphilis, the signs and symptoms of widespread infection begin to manifest themselves. It is popularly believed that the main affliction is of the skin, because that is what is most readily seen and diagnosed. However, syphilis is a systemic infection and, if the treponeme is looked for, it will be found to be affecting many different organs in the body, from the liver to the lungs and the brain to the bones.

There is a feeling of malaise, that is 'unwellness', on top of which may be specific symptoms due to the involvement of certain organs or parts of the body. There may be fever, loss of appetite and weight, and aches and pains in the muscles, joints, and bones. Over 75 per cent of people with secondary syphilis will have some form of rash, and about 50 per cent will have a generalized enlargement of the lymph glands. There will be spots or sores on the mucous membranes in one third of cases, and 10 per cent will have signs of involvement of other parts of the body including the eye, nervous system, bones, or internal organs.

Syphilis has long been labelled 'the great imitator' and there are only a few clues to prod the examining doctor into thinking of the correct diagnosis rather than some other condition. The rash may take one of several forms — it may mimic a host of rare and not so rare skin conditions. The first and perhaps most useful clue is that in the majority of cases the rash is non-irritating. It is also found on the palms of the hand and the soles of the feet, which are not sites commonly affected by other rashes. The rash may be barely visible, and may only be present for a few days, or it may be widespread and obvious and persist for many weeks.

Clearly, the specialists who see most cases are either venereologists or dermatologists, but many's the case of secondary syphilis that has been treated by a general practitioner or physician with a variety of ointments or creams to great effect — syphilis having the doctor-flattering attribute of 'getting better' whatever the treatment. It was this particular characteristic of syphilis, that both the primary sore and the secondary rash will go away after a certain period, that produced so many varied cures in the pre-antibiotic era. The best treatment in the nineteenth century was the one that did the least harm to the patient.

Case history. Philip H., a 35-year-old homosexual music arranger, was seen at the ENT department of a Midlands hospital with ringing in the ears. This 'tinnitus' is a symptom of several medical conditions, ranging from excess wax in the external ear to infection in the middle ear or direct involvement of the nerve responsible for hearing. Had a sexual history been taken at the time of his first visit, it would have emerged that, although he had a long-lasting and stable sexual relationship with one person, his partner was of a promiscuous nature and was known by Philip H. to have had several casual sexual encounters over the preceding year. As it was, all manner of sophisticated tests failed to reveal the cause of the tinnitus. Poor Philip was particularly bothered by this symptom because he had perfect pitch and being in the music business used to go over music in his mind most of his waking hours. The ringing in his ears happened to be a bare half tone below the key in which he hummed music to himself. When he was seen in the special department, after blood tests for syphilis, taken as a last resort, had turned out strongly positive, he remembered having noticed a sore on his penis some five months earlier but had not bothered with it as it was not painful and had gone away after a couple of weeks. He had not noticed any skin rash and was surprised to be told that his symptom was a direct result of syphilis affecting the auditory nerve. Within one week of

PLATE 5: Syphilis

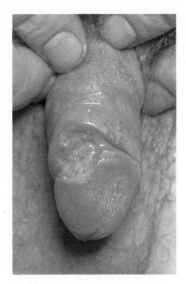

Primary chancre of penis

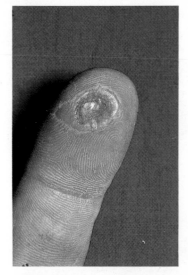

Primary chancre on finger

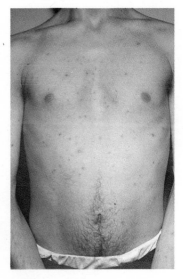

Secondary rash

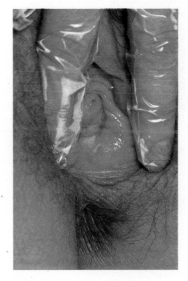

Primary chancre of vulva

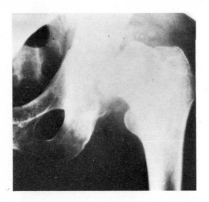

PLATE 6

Late Syphilis

Destruction of the hip joint

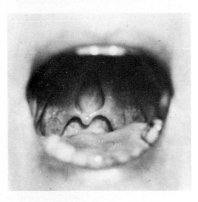

Perforation of palate

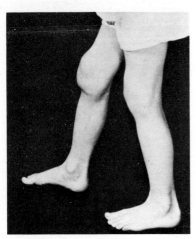

Destruction of knee joint

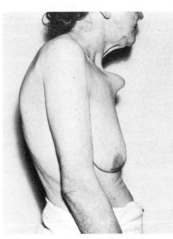

Aneurysm of aorta eroding through chest

starting penicillin treatment the ringing had gone and he was able to return to work.

Although this particular complication must be exceedingly rare, it bears out the point that syphilis is a multi-system disease and in the secondary stage can present in the most unlikely ways. There is evidence of asymptomatic involvement of the central nervous system in up to 20 per cent of cases with secondary syphilis but in the majority of these there will only be a transient headache, if anything, to signify this complication.

The eyes and the liver are sometimes involved late in the secondary stage, as are the joints and the covering of the bones. Like the central nervous system complications, however, they may be difficult to diagnose without the clues given by the coincidental involvement of the skin and mucous membranes.

After a period of some weeks without treatment, the rash and any other manifestations of secondary syphilis will regress and the disease enters the early latent stage. During this period, which lasts until the end of the second year after acquiring the infection, there will be no signs or symptoms of the disease, although infectious organisms are still present in the tissues. In a few cases the disease undergoes a recurrent phase when the manifestations of secondary syphilis are seen again. Needless to say, the lesions on the skin in the recurrent phase are still infectious.

In some cases of syphilis that have been treated, relapse may occur. This is probably a result of inadequate treatment and is more common in those who have been treated late on in the infectious stage. It is for this reason that patients are followed up for two years after treatment. It should be added that relapse is uncommon and is almost certainly less common than reinfection as a cause of reappearance of active syphilis.

Late syphilis

The late latent stage of syphilis, like the early latent stage, is an asymptomatic period when there is virtually no chance of the infection being passed on. Many people who have reached this stage in their infection can look forward to no further trouble from their disease and will probably die of old age or some other condition unrelated to their syphilis. Some, however, will go on to the tertiary or 'gummatous' stage and a few will go on to develop neurological or cardiovascular complications. All these complications are extremely rare these days in the United Kingdom, and what few cases there are tend to have acquired their infection in the thirties or forties, before widespread use of antibiotics brought the possibility of permanent cure.

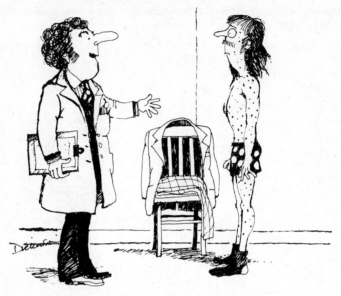

'Relax it's not syphilis, you've got smallpox.'

Tertiary syphilis

The lesion in this stage is known as the gumma. The pathological process responsible for the lesions is, as in early syphilis, an inflammation and blocking of the small arteries. Treponemes are difficult to find microscopically in these lesions, but if material from a gumma is injected into a rabbit, it will produce a syphilitic infection. The skin lesions, in contrast to those of secondary syphilis, are asymmetrical. Like the secondary lesions they may mimic other skin conditions and can be found on the surface of the skin, or sometimes as lumps or nodules beneath it. The mucous membranes may also be involved, and painless ulcers can be found in the mouth and throat. If the hard palate or septum of the nose are involved, the underlying bone is also affected and can be perforated. The tongue may be infiltrated by gummatous change, and this occasionally progresses through so-called 'leukoplakic' change to end in cancer of the tongue. Gummata are also found in the bones, muscles, and internal organs. It should be emphasized that all these complications are exceedingly rare in the Western world today.

Cardiovascular syphilis

Although reliable figures are difficult to obtain, some 10 per cent of patients with late, untreated syphilis will go on to develop syphilitic complications involving the heart and major blood-vessels. Three main complications may occur, separately or in combination.

Involvement of the valve of the aorta (the large main artery, emerging from the heart), can cause this valve to become inefficient, so that instead of closing fully after each pumping beat of the heart, it remains partly open, allowing a proportion of the blood to return to the heart instead of passing on round the body. Any great degree of such aortic valve incompetence will place an unacceptable work-load on the heart, with resulting heart failure. There are many other more common causes of aortic incompetence, including rheumatic fever, but cases of syphilitic aortic-valve disease still turn up from time to time in this country, albeit rarely.

The second complication is called coronary ostial stenosis. With this complication, the opening of the coronary arteries (which supply blood to the heart muscle itself) are involved by the syphilitic process. This causes a narrowing of the channel and diminishes the amount of blood that the coronary arteries can carry. When this happens, any excess demands on the heart, such as hard exercise, will result in a lack of oxygen in the heart muscle, and angina pectoris — typical cardiac pain — will result. Occasionally ostial stenosis leads to a full-blown heart attack.

The third important complication of cardiovascular syphilis is the development of aneurysms in the wall of the aorta or other major arteries. An aneurysm is a swelling or dilatation caused by a weakening in the wall of a blood-vessel. Syphilitic aneurysms most commonly occur in that part of the aorta which is found in the chest, but occasionally are found in the abdominal aorta. Syphilitic aneurysms cause most of their symptoms by pressure on surrounding structures in the chest.

Neurosyphilis

It has been mentioned that a proportion of patients with secondary syphilis will show evidence of involvement of the central nervous system, usually of the meninges (meningitis), the covering layers of the brain and spinal cord. Some, like Philip H., will develop symptoms, while the majority give and are given no indication that the disease has spread to the nervous system. A small proportion of patients with untreated syphilis will go on to develop brain or spinal cord complications many years after the original infection. Unlike cardiovascular syphilis, which is more common among Negroid races than Caucasian, neurosyphilis occurs more often in white patients.

If the cerebro-spinal fluid (CSF) is examined in cases of late latent syphilis, a proportion of cases will be shown to have abnormalities indicative of neurosyphilis when there are no overt signs or symptoms of this complication. Some, but not all, will go on to develop late complications.

These may result in malfunction of the cranial nerves with thrombosis of the arteries supplying blood to the brain. If this latter event occurs, the result may be difficult to distinguish from a stroke due to atheroma in these arteries. Syphilis of the brain tissue leads to progressive neurological deterioration known as *general paralysis of the insane* (GPI). A gradual diminution in mental faculties which is noticed by friends and relatives but not by the affected person is the first change. The memory is lost and judgement is impaired. The classical progression is then to delusions of grandeur with absurd claims of past and present achievements. More commonly, however, there is gradually increasing dementia with an overlying depression. Along with the mental deterioration comes a physical decline with fits, incontinence, difficulty with speech, and a degree of spastic paralysis.

When the spinal cord is involved a condition known as *tabes dorsalis* occurs. The main features of tabes are an inability to balance when the eyes are shut, numbness, and 'tingling' sensations, 'lightning pains', which are sharp, shooting pains, usually in the lower limbs, which may come and go in a short time or last for several days without remission. There may be bladder or bowel disturbances due to malfunction of the nerves supplying these functions. The sacral nerves which supply the genitalia are often involved in the disease process, and this may lead to sexual anaesthesia in the female and impotence in the male. The lack of sensory feedback may lead to severe arthritis in the joints involved, called, after the nineteenth-century French physician who described the changes, Charcot's arthropathy. Optic atropy, with its gradual deterioration in sight, complicates some 20 per cent of cases of tabes dorsalis.

Congenital syphilis

Syphilis can be acquired by the unborn foetus from its mother if she has the infection and there are treponemes circulating in the blood stream. There is no evidence that the father can pass the disease directly to the foetus without first infecting the mother. The likelihood of a syphilitic mother passing the infection on when she is pregnant diminishes the longer she has had the disease, and when she has been given an adequate course of anti-syphilitic treatment, there is no chance of her infecting her unborn child unless she herself becomes reinfected. Not only are the chances of the infection being passed on diminished with the length of the infection, but the severity of infection in the child also diminishes with time. Thus a mother with early infectious syphilis is likely either to miscarry or to give birth to a stillborn child. If she has early latent syphilis there is a 20 per cent chance that the child will be unaffected, and this figure rises to 70 per cent if the mother has late syphilis. The mode of infection is by the mother's blood, which contains treponemes. These can pass from the maternal circulation across the placenta.

In most countries it is customary to test the mother's blood for evidence of syphilis when she is first seen for antenatal care, and this one measure is probably responsible for the extreme rarity of cases of early congenital syphilis. The number of cases in England and Wales was 227 in 1950, 18 in 1960, and 12 in 1970. There remains the possibility that the pregnant mother may catch the infection after her first antenatal examination, or that she was incubating early syphilis and therefore had negative blood-tests when first seen.

Congenital syphilis is arbitrarily divided into early and late stages with the dividing line at two years of age. Rather like those adults with syphilis acquired from infected blood at transfusion or who have suffered an accidental inoculation from an infected syringe, the baby with congenital syphilis has no primary stage in the infection.

The baby may appear completely normal at birth or may be born with signs similar to those of adult secondary syphilis. There may be a generalized rash, widespread lymphadenopathy, and mucous membrane lesions. If these latter involve the nose and pharynx, this leads to 'snuffles' in which there is a profuse nasal discharge which may be bloodstained and is teeming with treponemes. The discharge may interfere with feeding and is highly infectious to anyone who comes into contact with it, apart from its mother. In addition to the skin lesions there may be involvement of the liver and spleen, the bones and eyes, and occasionally the central nervous system with a syphilitic meningitis.

In the majority of cases of *late* congenital syphilis the condition is in a latent phase, and it may be difficult to decide whether the infection is congenital or acquired. The most common late manifestation is interstitial keratitis in which the cornea of the eye gradually clouds over, rather like a cataract. There may be neurological involvement similar to that occurring in adult acquired syphilis, but the onset is, of course, at a much younger age. Late lesions of the bones and joints occur, and frequently a progressive deafness develops. Gummata may be found, particularly in the palate or nose. Cardio-vascular involvement is, however, extremely rare.

Certain so-called 'stigmata' are seen in congenital syphilis, and these are the residual scars and deformities of early infection. These stigmata are not invariable and many congenital syphilitics bear only positive blood tests as evidence of their congenital disease. Abnormalities of the teeth, known as Hutchinson's teeth, are sometimes found. The facial appearance may be diagnostic if the nasal infection was severe. The bridge of the nose is depressed with a 'saddle' appearance and the upper jaw may be small compared to the lower. This gives a typical 'bulldog' appearance. There may be small scars at the corners of the mouth known as 'rhagades' and there are sometimes deformed nails due to damage of the nail-bed.

The blood-tests

Whereas the diagnosis of early infectious syphilis can be made with a good degree of accuracy by identifying the treponeme with dark-ground examination of serum from a chancre or from the skin lesions of secondary infection, in latent or late syphilis, be it acquired or con-genital, the diagnosis depends on the finding of antibodies to the infec-tion in the blood. Virtually all infections, be they sexually transmitted or not, provoke the formation of antibodies, some of which can be found circulating in the blood-stream. In some infections these anti-bodies are effective as preventers of further infection by the same organism. This is why it is unusual to catch measles or chicken-pox more than once, and why immunization and vaccination are effective in preventing various diseases. Sadly, with syphilis, the measurable increases in the blood levels of circulating antibodies do not reflect any useful level of protection against repeated infection. What they can do, however, is to help the physician come to a diagnosis and even measure the effect of treatment on the infection.

The serological tests for syphilis (STS) fall into two categories. The non-specific or 'reagin' tests, exemplified by the Wasserman reaction (WR), and the specific tests of which the important ones are the *Trepo-nema pallidum* immobilization test (TPI), the *Treponema pallidum* haemagglutination test (TPHA), and the fluorescent treponemal anti-body test (FTA). The reagin tests, which were the first tests to become widely available, are still in common use. They have the advantage that they are easy to perform, they are cheap, and their degree of positivity varies *pari passu* with the state of the infection. The most common test of this sort to be performed is the Venereal Disease Reference Lab-oratory test (VDRL). This test is very strongly positive when there is active infection and becomes negative, or nearly so, when the infection has been adequately treated. It can thus be used to monitor the effects of treatment. It will also detect reinfection when it has occurred. The main drawback with the VDRL and other reagin tests is that they may become positive with conditions other than treponemal infection. These 'biological false-positive' reactions have many causes, including many virus diseases, vaccinations, and some other generalized diseases.

The specific tests, on the other hand, very rarely give false-positive reactions, but are, like the reagin tests, unable to distinguish between syphilis and the other, non-venereal, treponemal diseases. They also tend to remain positive for a very long time, if not indefinitely, unless the infection has been treated in the very early stages. The ideal screening system, such as might be used in antenatal clinics should utilize one of each sort of test so that a combination of sensitivity with selectivity can be obtained.

Treatment

Since the discovery of penicillin, the treatment of syphilis has been revolutionized. When first introduced, it was customary to give daily injections for periods of ten to twenty days, and this is still the practice in many clinics both in this country and elsewhere in the world. This treatment is highly effective but smacks a little of a rather punitive approach to the patient now that long-acting penicillins are available which only need to be given once or twice a week. There is a good case these days for treatment of syphilis to be with these more modern forms of penicillin.

The treponeme, unlike the gonococcus, has shown no sign of developing resistance to penicillin or any other antibiotics and, once diagnosed, is easy to eradicate. All forms of early syphilis can be completely cured, and some of the later manifestations can be markedly improved, or, at least, the progression of the disease can be arrested. Several other antibiotics can be used in the treatment of syphilis, to good effect, but penicillin remains the drug of choice.

The *Jarisch–Herxheimer* reaction, usually shortened to the 'Herxheimer' reaction, follows the initial dose of treatment of syphilis in a proportion of cases. It probably results from the break-up of treponemes in response to the penicillin, with release of substances into the bloodstream and locally which have an inflammatory potential. There is usually a flu-like episode lasting 12 to 24 hours with headache, aches and pains in the muscles and joints, and fever. The reaction occurs most frequently in cases of early infectious syphilis when 50 per cent or more patients will notice some upset or other. Apart from these systemic effects, there may be a quite marked local inflammation with swelling and white-cell infiltration. This may lead to catastrophic results in a few cases of late syphilis when the cardiovascular or nervous systems are involved. If, for instance the openings of the coronary arteries are involved by the syphilitic process, the swelling of the tissues after treatment may lead to blockage and sudden death. Luckily, the Herxheimer reaction is less common in late syphilis, but it is still usual to try to lessen the chances of adverse reaction by giving anti-inflammatory steroid tablets before treatment begins.

It is usual to follow patients who have been diagnosed and treated for syphilis for a period of two years to make sure that the treatment is effective and that relapse does not occur. This involves the patient's attending for repeat blood-tests. There is evidence that following the start of treatment the lesions of primary or secondary syphilis are free of active treponemes within 48 hours, although it would be a brave person who took this to mean that intercourse was safe so soon after starting treatment.

9

The infestations

There are many arthropods associated with human disease, ranging from the larvae of certain flies such as the 'Congo maggot' which are obligatory tissue parasites and eat away the flesh of an infested person, to the scorpion whose sting can cause serious illness and in some cases, particularly children, even death. Fleas, ticks, and spiders of various kinds are associated with disease either directly as a result of their bites or because they act as vectors of infections such as typhus and the relapsing fevers. Now, while it would be rash to claim that cochliomyasis (infestation with the 'screw worm fly') was *never* sexually transmitted, like most of the other arthropod-linked disorders, such an occurrence must be exceedingly uncommon.

There are two infestations that are commonly transmitted in this way although there is no absolute necessity for this mode of transmission. These are infestation with *Phthirus pubis* and *Sarcoptes scabiei*.

Phthirus pubis

The pubic or 'crab' louse is one of three members of the family Pediculidae, a sub-group of the Anoplura or sucking lice, to be of clinical interest to men. *Pediculus humanus corporis*, the body louse, and *Pediculus homanus capitis*, the head louse, share with *Phthirus pubis* three pairs of legs, a predilection for man or the higher apes, and a dependence on fresh blood, to which they must have access at least twice a day. The body louse may lay its eggs in clothing or bedding, while the head louse, like the crab louse, cements its eggs on to hairs forming 'nits', which are the size of a pin-head and can just be made out with the naked eye. The pubic louse is broader than it is long and the four hind legs are equipped with claws with which it hangs on to the pubic hairs. This gives it a passing resemblance to a crab, with which it shares an inability to raise itself significantly above any flat surface on which it finds itself, giving the lie to that universally popular, but inaccurate, graffito, 'Please to stand upon the seat, the crabs in here can jump six feet'.

In addition to the three pairs of legs and four pairs of feet which are found behind the legs, the crab louse is equipped with sensory antennae and eyes. The former allow the louse to detect the smell of man. There are tactile hairs which enable the louse to appreciate the type of surface it is on. Lice are very temperature-sensitive and will leave a body which is running a fever.

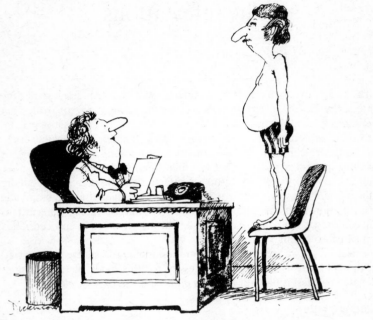

'I think the graffito was right in your case, Mr Smith.'

Pubic lice are usually confined to the pubic and anal areas, although, in very hairy people, they may be found on the chest and in the axillary hair. Very occasionally, they can be found on the eyelashes and eyebrows, but they are said never to be found higher than that. The reason that they stick almost exclusively to the pubic region is, appropriately, a sexual one. Pubic hairs are further apart than hairs elsewhere on the body and, in particular, than the hairs of the head. For successful coitus to take place, the male and female lice each grab two adjacent hairs with both pairs of rear legs, front to front. This juxtaposition is impossible if the hairs are too close together, as on the scalp.

The male pubic louse has a rather more pointed tail than the female and is smaller and more active. There are usually more females than males present on an infested person and the males are relatively promiscuous, mating frequently. The female may lay up to 50 eggs during its lifetime and averages perhaps three eggs per day. To lay an egg, the female grasps a hair and deposits some 'cement' which is extruded on to a hair just before the egg is laid. The cement is very powerful and will not be removed by hot water, soaps, or detergents.

Symptoms and signs of pubic louse infestation

It is difficult to establish an exact incubation period for genital louse infection but various authorities agree that the average time between acquiring and noticing the lice is about one month. Not all infested people will develop symptoms, and those who do may not ascribe their itching to the presence of crabs in the pubic area. In only one in four cases has the patient actually seen the crab lice. The main symptom is that of itching which occurs mostly at night. Although the itching may be due to the movement of the louse over the skin, it only moves a maximum of six inches per day, and it is more likely that an allergic reaction is set up to the lice themselves or to their faeces. This would explain why most people fail to develop symptoms right at the beginning of the infestation. Itching can be intense, and there may be a visible rash, which can become secondarily infected by bacteria. Faintly bluish spots may develop at the site of a louse bite and persist for several days.

About two millimetres across, the crab louse is often difficult to see. It will tend to lie doggo in the light and, because it is flat, it can easily be mistaken for a small mole on the skin. They can be very difficult to prise away from the hairs to which they are attached. Once detached, they can be seen moving very slowly away. Their natural colour is brown, but after feeding, when they may increase their body weight by a third, they take on a redder tinge. The nits, also brown in colour, can be seen attached to the pubic hair, and examination with a magnifying glass will distinguish those containing a developing larva, which takes a week before it leaves the egg, from those which have already been vacated.

If there is infestation of the eyelashes or eyebrows, there may be a marked blepharitis, inflammation around the eye, which can be difficult to diagnose and is resistant to treatment until the correct diagnosis is made. Careful examination will reveal the tell-tale nits attached to the hairs.

As Virtues's *Household physician* (1924) so succinctly puts it, 'the main object in the treatment of these filthy diseases is the destruction of the parasite . . . strict cleanliness of the person is a *sine qua non* . . . the remedies usually employed are the mercurials, sulphur, carbolic acid, tobacco, etc.'

The adult lice can be removed along with the nits by painstakingly using a pair of tweezers and a magnifying glass. Shaving the pubic hair is an alternative 'physical' approach, but nowadays there are several preparations on the market which have the desired effect rather more easily. Dichloro-diphenyl trichlorethane, dicophane or DDT, was the first really specific agent to become available and is is still effective against the adult lice, although there is evidence of the development of resistance. Unfortunately, it has no effect on the larval stage in the eggs and further applications may need to be given to cope with the larvae as they hatch. In spite of Virtues's dogma, cleanliness is neither essential nor effective against an established infestation, and gamma-benzene hexachloride or benzyl benzoate are preferable and more effective than either carbolic acid or tobacco.

One application of the benzene derivatives will kill all the adult lice and all the developing larvae as well. Although the young lice inside the eggs are killed by this application, the nits will remain attached to the hairs firmly and a fine-toothed comb may be needed to detach them.

As with other sexually transmitted infections, it should be remembered that any sexual partners will need to be closely examined and treated if necessary. Although the mode of transmission is predominantly a sexual one, sharing a bed platonically with an infested person can be the cause. *Phthirus pubis* is unable to survive away from the human host for more than 24 hours and it is readily killed by temperatures over 50 °C. One is unlikely to catch the infection from sleeping in a bed previously occupied by an infested person and there is no need, as there is when dealing with body lice, to take special care with clothing and bed linen.

Two out of every five people with crab lice will have some other form of sexually transmitted disease, and both doctors and patients should be aware of this and be on the lookout for other signs and symptoms.

Sarcoptes scabiei

The causative organism of scabies is a mite, and as such a member of the class Arachnida, which includes the spiders and scorpions. They have eight legs. There are many different varieties of scabetic mite infesting various mammals, and, although the mites from different animals appear to be similar, they are probably species specific because infestation by the mite from domestic animals does not 'take' in the human and dies out after a few weeks. People who come into frequent contact with domestic animals may become transiently infected but the symptoms do not last for any appreciable period.

Unlike the crab louse, the mite of scabies lays its eggs under the skin surface, and to do this it needs to burrow through the thick outer layer of the skin. The eggs, which are the same size as the adult male mite, take 3 to 4 days to hatch into the three-legged larva. The larva moults to give rise to the four-legged nymph, which, after five more days, becomes the adult mite. The adult female, initially the same size as the male, becomes twice as large after fertilization as the ovaries swell up with developing eggs.

There are two sets of front legs, which end in what look like suckers. The two pairs of rear legs end in bristles. There is no head as such, but instead there is a small protrubrance at the front end, which contains the mouth parts.

Although, at less than ½ mm in length, it is smaller than the crab louse, it appears more willing to move, and a mite has been timed at one inch per minute.

It may be that only one fertilized female is needed to infect a new victim. It takes about one hour for the mite to bury itself in the skin. After selecting a suitable site, the mite will use its mouth parts and its four front legs. These latter are equipped with sharp joints above the suckers and are used in a 'sawing' motion to cut through the skin.

Once ensconced in her burrow, the female mite will soon begin to lay eggs, which accumulate behind her at the rate of three or four a day. Unless she is scratched out, the adult female will remain in her burrow until she dies. If scratching by the human host removes the roof of the burrow, the mite will wander away until it finds another suitable site. When the nymphs are hatched into young males and females, they each make a shallow burrow from which they emerge at night to search for a mate. The male does not live as long as the female, and this would explain the relative paucity of males.

The mite of scabies has a particular preference for certain sites on the body, and, if placed away from one of these favoured places, will make its way to a more satisfactory area. The genital region, wrists, and finger webs are the most commonly affected sites, followed by the elbows, feet, buttocks, armpits, and breasts, particularly around the nipples. The average number of mites found in a case of scabies is about ten. This is considerably less than the numbers found in the animal equivalent, sarcoptic mange, where literally thousands of mites are to be found. Occasionally such a massive infestation occurs in man, when it goes by the name of crusted or Norwegian scabies.

It is not for nothing that scabies is commonly known as *the itch*. The itch is not a painful one and James I is said to have claimed that the itch was fitted only for kings, so exquisite was the enjoyment of scratching. Most people suffering from scabies would gladly donate their symptoms to royalty, or anyone else for that matter. The itching, which is worse at night, particularly affects areas where the skin is loose, and the armpits, lower abdomen, buttocks, and thighs seem to suffer the most. It may become intolerable and make sleep impossible. Because of the scratching that is provoked, the burrows of the mite and the surrounding skin become excoriated and bacterial infection may supervene. The rash in such cases may not look at all like simple uncomplicated scabies.

Although the night-time itching has been put down to the nocturnal habits of the mite, it is interesting that for the first few weeks of infestation, when the mites are presumably just as active, there are often no symptoms at all. When the itching does begin it is probably because an allergic or sensitivity reaction has been set up. Whether it is to the mite or its faeces that the victim becomes sensitive, once itching has started the discomfort gets progressively worse. This allergic reaction explains why, after successful treatment of the infection, itching may continue for some weeks because of the dead remains of the mite persisting under the skin.

The burrow caused by *Sarcoptes scabiei* can be recognized as a thin line, not unlike a small splinter, in one of the sites which the mite is known to favour. Sometimes, in a person who has become sensitized, there may be small vesicles in the skin which release a clear fluid when ruptured after scratching.

If a further infection occurs in someone who has already suffered from scabies, the course of events may be very different. Itching will begin within an hour or so of the invasion, and the vigorous scratching induced may well abort the attack. If, however, there is a constant flow of parasites from an infected sleeping partner, say, then previous sensitization will be unable to prevent further infection.

Before getting on to the commonest mode of transmission of scabies, it will be worth while stressing the ways it is *not* transmitted. Towels, flannels, lavatories, and seats in buses and trains are not incriminated. Although it is theoretically possible to catch scabies by sleeping in a bed previously occupied by a sufferer from scabies, the chances are extremely remote. Prolonged contact with someone who has scabies is the most likely method of transmission. When it occurs, as it often does, in young children, it may have been passed on by holding hands, but the most frequent opportunity for transmission is afforded by the close proximity of sharing a bed. Sexual intercourse does not have to take place, more important is prolonged, warm, close contact.

The same products are used for treating scabies as are used for pubic lice. In the case of scabies, however, the lotion should be carefully applied over the whole body surface from the neck downwards. If this is done efficiently no further treatment will be necessary. Because, for reasons mentioned earlier, the itching may persist for some time, and just in case the first application was not exhaustive, it is quite common to advise a second treatment one week after the first. There should not be any need for this. It is obviously important to check all other members of a household and make sure that any other infested people are treated. There is no need to launder bedding or sterilize clothing.

10

The tropical diseases

There are two groups of tropical diseases of importance; those that are sexually transmitted – chancroid, granuloma inguinale, and lympho-granuloma venereum, and those that, although passed on in a non-sexual fashion, are closely related to syphilis and may be confused with it. These include yaws, bejel, and pinta.

Chancroid

Chancroid, also called soft sore, soft chancre, and 'ulcus molle', is a disease of world-wide distribution but is seen only rarely in temperate climates and is uncommon in Western Europe or North America and, when it has been diagnosed, it has usually been imported from warmer countries. Only 68 cases were seen in England in 1976 and these were mostly seen in or near ports. Its name implies similarity with the primary sore of syphilis but it is ill-named, for the only feature in common with syphilis is the presence of genital ulceration and by this criterion there are at least six other conditions that could be equally well so labelled.

It is caused by a bacterium *Haemophilus ducreyi*, which is often very difficult to grow in the laboratory and correspondingly hard to find in the lesions themselves. This, coupled with its comparative rarity in the Western world, has lead some of the more cynical amongst physicians to doubt its very existence, and to suggest that it is really a collection of ulcerative genital conditions including herpes and trauma. The enormous variety in the clinical descriptions of the primary sores, from 'dwarf' to 'giant', 'transient' to 'phagedenic' (destructive of tissue), and 'follicular' to 'papular' might be taken as lending a little indirect support for this heresy. Be that as it may, chancroid is diagnosed and treated with frequency in endemic areas where it has been described as a disease of the socially unenlightened and the economically unfortunate. If this is so, then it is unique among sexually transmitted diseases as a respecter of social class. It is disproportionately uncommon among women, and some authorities believe this is due to its producing a carrier state in females.

Usually within a week of contracting the disease, ulcers develop on

91

the genitalia. Multiple rather than single ulcers are the rule, in contra-distinction to syphilis. The ulcers are acutely painful, with soft bases unlike the thickened painless ulcer of syphilis. Spread of the ulcers can occur by auto-inoculation and rarely the spread may be such as to cause gangrene of the penis. As with Herpes genitalis, the main symptom in the woman is pain due to the flow of urine over the lesions. The infec-tion spreads via the lymphatic vessels to the lymph nodes of the groin where there is usually a one-sided swelling, called the inflammatory bubo. This swelling enlarges, becomes very painful, and, if untreated, will eventually break down and discharge pus.

Treatment is with broad-spectrum antibiotics or sulphonamides. As with all the sexually transmitted diseases, the possibility of other con-current infection must be considered and excluded.

Lymphogranuloma venereum (LGV)

At least with this disease there is no doubt as to its existence, although the causative organism is as difficult to grow and identify as that of chancroid.

Like chancroid, LGV is common in tropical and sub-tropical climates and uncommon in temperate ones, such cases as are seen being imported into this country. The causative organism, like that responsible for many cases of non-specific infection, is a member of the chlamydia group. The incubation period is usually between one and two weeks, although longer periods have been described. As its name implies, the infection attacks the lymphatic system, and, although the disease is localized rather than systemic, it can produce considerable destruction of tissue near the genitalia, particularly in women, if allowed to continue un-treated for any length of time.

In men the primary lesion of LGV is a small ulcer or spot, which appears on the shaft or glans penis. It is often so insignificant that it is either ignored by the patient or passed off as a 'pimple'. In half the cases there is no history of a primary lesion at all. The primary lesion is followed, after an interval of one to four weeks, by the appearance of swollen lymph nodes on one or both sides of the groin. The glands become matted together and very painful to the touch. There is usually a clearly seen demarcation between upper and lower sausage-shaped groups of glands, which has aptly been named the 'sign of the groove'. The inguinal swelling (or 'bubo') continues to enlarge and eventually forms abscesses which break down and discharge on to the skin. Some-times, if on the right side, the abdominal pain associated with LGV may be mistaken for acute appendicitis.

There may be a generalized constitutional upset with fever, headache, loss of appetite and weight, and joint pains. If untreated, recovery occurs after a few weeks, but discharging abscesses may remain in the groin.

In women it is rare for either the patient or the examining doctor to notice a primary lesion, and the next stage, that of the inguinal bubo, is usually less marked than in men. This is because the drainage of the genital region in women is more often to groups of lymph glands in the pelvis, and their involvement is not likely to be obvious. Infection in these nodes may lead to backache. This relative lack of symptoms combined with the involvement of internal lymph nodes probably explains why the complications of LGV are both more common and more serious in women.

Because the disease affects the lymph channels and glands, there is disruption of the normal fluid drainage from the genital area. The result of this is the development of chronic lymphatic oedema, due to accumulation of fluid, and eventually to elephantiasis, which is irreversible enlargement. This complication is rare in men but causes a gross swelling of the vulva in females, called esthiomene. The swelling may extend from the clitoris to the anus. Wart-like growths may occur on the skin. When oedema of the male genitalia occurs, it may give rise to the intriguingly-named 'saxophone penis'.

Because of the close proximity of the vagina to the rectum, women are more prone to suffer the other important late complications of LGV, the so-called ano-rectal syndrome, in which the infective and inflammatory processes involve the lower bowel. These complications are rare in males but have been described in male homosexuals. Very rarely, malignant change may occur resulting in cancer of the bowel or genitalia.

The diagnoses of early infection in the male and late infection in the female may be suggested by the clinical findings, the groove sign being very characteristic in the early stages. It may be possible to grow the causative organism in the laboratory and, failing that, it is often possible to demonstrate measurable increases in specific antibodies in the blood.

The condition is treated with sulphonamides or tetracyclines and the inguinal bubo may be aspirated or drained before it bursts. Surgical removal of the redundant tissue in cases of esthiomene may be necessary and the intestinal obstruction in the ano-rectal syndrome may require colostomy.

Granuloma inguinale

Like chancroid and lymphogranuloma venereum, granuloma inguinale is not commonly seen in the United Kingdom, there being only sixteen cases reported in 1976. Some doubt has been expressed about the method of spread of this disease since it is by no means always found in the sexual partners of infected individuals. It is certainly of low contagiousness and there is a possibility that the condition follows auto-infection from the bowel, where the causative organism can be found.

Over 60 per cent of cases occur in males, and it is much more common among the Negro races than Caucasians, although this may reflect the areas where it is endemic rather than any racial predilection. Granuloma inguinale is endemic in India and cases are also seen in Africa, the West Indies, and the southern states of America.

It is caused by a bacterium called *Donovania granulomatis*. This bacterium can be found in the skin lesions and has the appearance of a safety-pin when visualized under the microscope. It has not been possible to pass the disease on to animals or to human volunteers by inoculation of the organism.

The incubation period is not accurately known, but may be as much as two months. The initial lesion starts as a small papule or vesicle, which ulcerates and spreads leaving a raised, velvety reddened area, which bleeds easily. The lesions are not confined to the genitalia, although they are most often found there, but are also seen on the thighs, perineum, and buttocks. There is no associated enlargement of lymph nodes, but small nodules under the surface of the skin in the groin may give rise to a 'pseudo-bubo'. Spread is slow and extension may take place over a period of months, even years. Secondary infection with other bacteria sometimes occurs and there may be widespread tissue destruction leading to loss of the penis in some cases. Scarring can occur and elephantiasis of the genitalia has been described, as has malignant change in late lesions, leading to carcinoma of the genitalia.

The bacterium is difficult to grow and it may be necessary to biopsy one of the lesions to come to the diagnosis.

Tropical treponematoses

Throughout the world there exist diseases caused by treponemes that are to all intents and purposes identical to *Treponema pallidum* yet which are not transmitted sexually and, in some cases, may co-exist with syphilis in the community. There are many clinical features in common among these treponematoses and some of them appear to go through similar stages and periods of latency. Whether the organisms responsible are in fact identical, and it is local factors that give the difference in clinical manifestations, or whether these diseases are examples of adaptive, divergent evolution, is not yet worked out. The reason for interest in these diseases stems from the massive emigration from countries where they are endemic to others where syphilis is the only or principal treponemal infection. Since the non-venereal treponematoses provoke identical antibody responses to those found in syphilis, problems arise in deciding whether such positive blood tests reflect, say, latent syphilis, or simply past infection by a non-venereal treponematosis in the country of origin.

Such difficulties are experienced in many countries in Europe with significant immigrant populations from the West Indies, in the United States, and in Australia and New Zealand. In practice it may be possible to make an enlightened guess as to the origin and type of infection involved, but in very few cases can the physician be one hundred per cent sure of his diagnosis.

Yaws. This disease occurs in tropical climes and used to be endemic in parts of Africa, South America, the Indian sub-continent, Indonesia, Australia, and the West Indies. The causative organism is called *Treponema pertenue*, and it is the same size, shape, and appearance as *Treponema pallidum*. It moves under the microscope with an identical corkscrew, bending motion. It is not sexually transmitted (although, like chicken pox or measles, it could be) and is usually acquired in early childhood by direct contact with an infected child. The site of the primary lesion, often referred to as the 'mother yaw', is on the leg in the majority of cases and, like the primary sore of syphilis, is painless unless there is other bacterial infection. If the primary lesion occurs on the sole of the foot it is known as a 'crab-yaw' because of the gait it induces. There is usually a painless swelling of the lymph glands which drain the area of the primary sore.

Some weeks after the appearance of the primary lesion, a secondary rash is seen, which is equivalent to that seen in secondary syphilis. Involvement of the covering of the bones may follow, and then the disease enters a latent phase. After five or ten years some cases will progress to a 'late' stage which is roughly equivalent to the tertiary, gummatous stage in syphilis. Bones and joints may be affected and if the process involves the nose and palate, a destructive, mutilating condition called *gangosa* occurs. Rarely, the central nervous system may be involved. It is considered unlikely that the disease can be transmitted to the foetus *in utero*. When a putative diagnosis of yaws is made in someone from an endemic area, on the strength of positive treponemal blood tests, it is customary to give a course of penicillin which would be adequate to treat latent syphilis should this have been the cause of the positive STS.

Bejel. Bejel, known locally as *firzal* and *loath* in the Middle East, and as *dichuchwa* in Botswana, usually presents in the secondary stage when skin lesions and mucous membrane lesions are seen. The disease may affect the larynx and bones, causing hoarseness and bone pains. Most infections occur in childhood, although it is said that those adults who have escaped infection when young may be infected by their own children, a reversal of roles from congenital syphilis.

The late manifestations involving the nervous and cardiovascular systems seen in syphilis do not occur and there seems to be no risk of passing on the infection to the unborn child. As with yaws, penicillin is the treatment of choice.

Pinta. This is the least damaging of the endemic treponematoses. It is found in Central and South America and, like yaws, is passed on in childhood. The primary lesion is known as a 'pintid' and appears, after an incubation period of some months, often on the legs. A secondary stage follows after a few months and manifests itself by a rash on the face and body. The destructive lesions seen in yaws do not occur, however, and bone lesions seldom cause trouble. Pinta (mal de pinto, carate) is caused by *Treponema careatum* which, like all the others, is indistinguishable from *Treponema pallidum*. Penicillin is used in treatment.

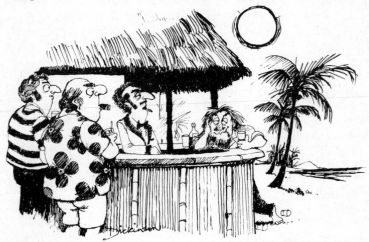

'Tragic! – brilliant physician, but people would keep saying "What's yaws Doc?"'

Endemic syphilis. Where the incidence of syphilis exceeds a certain high level, the disease becomes endemic and transmission may occur regularly in a non-sexual context. Such a situation existed in the Bosnian area of Yugoslavia around the time of the Second World War. Infection commonly occurs in children and infants, and the clinical progression of the disease is similar to syphilis when it is seen in the sporadic form; the late manifestations, however, tend to be seen at a much younger age. Congenital syphilis is rare in this situation because, by the time women get to child-bearing age, the disease has entered the late stage when transmission to the foetus is unlikely.

Following an intensive campaign by the World Health Organization, when mass injections of penicillin were given to everyone at risk, this form of syphilis has been eradicated in Yugoslavia. Similar campaigns have been waged in areas affected by other endemic treponematoses with considerable, if not equal, success.

11

The clinic

In the United Kingdom, in contrast to anywhere else in the world, the majority of cases of sexually transmitted disease are seen in clinics staffed by specialists trained particularly to deal with these problems. There has long been a tradition of separating these 'special' clinics from the rest of the hospital, and many of them still go under euphemistic titles such as 'Martha and Luke' clinic, James Pringle House, or 'Lydia' clinic. This geographical separation and disguised label reflects the old-fashioned and long-standing shame and stigma attached to all sexual matters, but in particular to the venereal diseases. It was felt that VD was naturally confined to the unwashed, unkempt, and morally barren, and, when occasionally seen in the better class of person, resulted from some supreme temptation that had been put before them, for indulgence in whose pleasures they could hardly be blamed. Anyway, if such a well-bred person was unlucky enough to be afflicted with one of these ailments, he was more likely to consult some understanding physician privately; and so it was largely the dirty and damned who attended the special clinics. It was obviously imperative that they should not mix with all the other nice clean patients attending the hospital with nice clean diseases.

The attitude that patients with sexually transmitted diseases are somehow different and decidedly inferior to the other members of the human race is still prevalent outside the medical profession, and, sadly, to a certain extent inside it. The message about acquisition of sexually transmitted diseases is a simple one. Every time that sexual intercourse takes place with a new partner there is a risk that some disease will be passed on from one to the other and, with rare exceptions, there is no way of telling, by simply looking at a person, whether they have an infection or not. There are obviously certain groups of people from whom there is a greater risk of catching a disease just as there are certain areas of the world where the prevalence of diseases is higher than others, but, wherever you are, it is the change of sexual partner that is the crucial risk-producing move. The more often that this happens, the more likely is any individual to acquire infection. The one-night stand is an obvious high-risk adventure and the question should be asked, 'Do I find myself in bed with this person because I am the most attractive/vivacious/brawny/amusing person that he/she has ever met or, if that is not true, what was he/she doing last night, and the night before, and the night before? And with whom?'; for the risk of catching VD can be directly related to the number of partner switches that take place. Not just yours, but those of your sexual partner as well. Because sexual adventures or misadventures are not the prerogative of the dirty, thick, and ill-educated, a representative cross-section of society will be found attending a typical clinic, including barristers and barmaids, doorkeepers and doctors. Nor are worries, fears, and guilt feelings the prerogative of the clean and educated and, what is more important, nor are all symptoms and signs referable to the genitalia the result of syphilis, or gonorrhoea, or even other, minor sexually transmitted diseases.

Figures from all the clinics in England and Wales in 1976 showed that only 16 per cent of attendances were by patients with venereal disease, as statutorily defined, and only a further 40 per cent had infections that were definitely sexually transmitted. Over 40 per cent of patients had other problems ranging from the clinically serious (rare) to the medically less important (more common). The latter category includes patients with cystitis, the urethral syndrome, vaginal discharge, sexual and contraceptive problems, and a sizeable minority who had nothing wrong with them at all. This broad spectrum of the work-load was one of the main reasons for changing the name of the specialty from venereology to genito-urinary medicine. The new name reflects more accurately the scope of the specialty, defines better the range of problems dealt with, and, most importantly, removes what was felt by many people to be an automatic stigma acquired by visiting the VD clinic.

In 1974 the Department of Health and Social Security published a short pamphlet entitled *Special treatment clinics – a design guide*. Considerable thought obviously went into the preparation of the recommendations, and clinics opened or planned since that time have largely followed the guidelines. Stating that clinics should have a close relationship with general out-patient departments, it goes on to suggest that, where ground-floor accommodation is unavailable, consideration should be given to allocating space at first-floor level, commenting, with rare insight, that this possibility arises because almost all the patients visiting the clinic will be ambulant.

Apart from giving advice on the size of accommodation, it lays down guidelines for the construction of consulting rooms and examination cubicles, with particular emphasis on sound insulation and the maintenance of confidentiality. It is pointed out that fluorescent lighting in clinical areas should be of a recommended type having colour rendering properties with which the decorative finishes in such areas must also be compatible. Nothing has been left out, from the temperature in the staff locker room (at 16 °C, 5 °C less than that in the examination rooms) to the number of changes of air per hour in the patients' lavatories (two!).

Clinics vary in size and in the percentages of different problems with which they deal, depending on where they are situated, and the characteristics of the local population that they serve. Thus in university towns and cities, there is often comparatively little gonorrhoea compared with the large urban areas, where shifting populations seem to be one of the reasons for an increased prevalence of the venereal diseases.

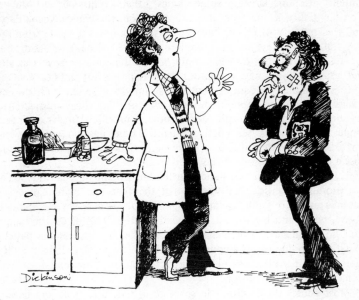

'I'm afraid that the clinic doesn't deal with injuries inflicted by irate wives.'

One of the great advantages of the clinic is that, unlike other out-patient departments, apart from the casualty department, no referral letter from a general practitioner is required. Although some patients do attend with a letter from their GP, many prefer to come directly to the clinic, as this saves time and possible embarrassment if they would rather that their family doctor didn't know about the particular problem. It is the general rule that the patient's own doctor will only be informed of the results of tests if the patient specifically requests it.

There are many different people who contribute to the efficient running of a clinic, including nurses, technicians, social workers, contact-tracers, doctors, and, the person who makes the first contact with a patient, the receptionist, whose contribution to the well-running of the department is of particular importance. If it has taken two weeks of nail-biting finally to pluck up courage to visit a clinic, only to be greeted by an unsympathetic or gruff receptionist, who demands details you had not expected to have to give in a loud voice, the temptation to cut and run may be overwhelming. Such an experience is, happily, rare.

Although some clinics still refer to their patient by number, most have now adopted the more human approach of calling people by their names. It is usual to ask for the age, address, and telephone number of patients attending and, in some clinics, other details may be sought. Confidentiality is the most important word in the clinic's vocabulary, and the majority of clinics have their own case-notes separate from the hospital notes. These are also stored in a different place. When addresses are required, these are needed only in case the clinic discovers an important infection a day or so after the patient has left and needs to get in touch in a hurry. Requests that letters should not be sent to the home address or that the telephone should not be used are always respected.

Some patients are, in spite of reassurance, unwilling to give their real names and in these cases a fictitious name is quite in order, with the one proviso that an attempt should be made to remember the false name in case a further visit should be needed.

It is important that all patients attending a clinic have confidence in the promised confidentiality, and that they can rest assured that this extends even to family relationships. Husbands and wives, sons and lovers, wives and boy-friends, husbands and girl-friends can be happy that no details will be released to their other half unless the patient specifically requests it. Of course, not all who attend a clinic have guilty secrets, and it is often useful for the doctor and both the sexual partners to have a joint consultation.

Most clinics divide either in space or in time into male and female sessions. In the larger clinics the two may run concurrently, in the smaller they may be held at different times during the week. I shall deal with a typical sequence of events for a man and a woman attending a clinic for the first time, for a check-up.

A female attendance

After registering with the receptionist, a set of case-notes is made out, and these are then sent through to the doctor who will be doing the interviewing and the examination. The delay between this booking-in and being seen by the doctor varies from day to day, from hour to hour, and from clinic to clinic. Most clinics provide an 'all-comers' service throughout clinic opening hours with no need to make an appointment. In a few clinics there is an appointments system which at least ensures that the patient is seen when he or she expects to be seen, but there may be delays in getting an appointment. Rather like the systems employed by general practitioners, there are advantages and disadvantages to both methods, with patients perhaps preferring the former system and being prepared to put up with a long delay once in the clinic to a worried wait of two or three days.

Because of the nature of the problems dealt with by departments of genito-urinary medicine, the questions asked by the doctor at the interview tend to be of an intimate nature. It should be remembered that it is not idle curiosity that prompts them. As a rule, the examining doctor will be well experienced in dealing with sexual symptoms and problems, and most patients find that they can talk about matters which would be difficult to discuss outside the clinic atmosphere and might even cause embarrassment if raised with their general practitioner. Details of recent sexual activity, when and with whom, are always important, even when there seems to be little likelihood of there being a sexually transmitted disease. Methods of contraception and details of the menstrual cycle — whether it has altered in any way, how regular it is — will be asked, and also details of the symptoms, if any, that prompted attendance. The doctor will want to know if the sexual partner has any symptoms and in particular whether he, too, has attended a clinic and, if so, what the diagnosis was and whether any treatment was given.

Any relevant past history of genital or urinary-tract problems should be mentioned, and also any sexual problems, such as pain on intercourse, decreased sex drive, or diminished satisfaction with the sexual act itself. Most people regard the sex act as a uniquely personal activity and find difficulty in imagining that anyone else could be suffering from the same problems as themselves. There may develop a fear that they are uniquely abnormal or that their sexual practices are uniquely unnatural.

After the interview with the doctor there may be a short wait before the examination itself begins. It is the prospect of this examination that seems to fill many women with terror, even to the point at which it provides the reason for putting off attendance. Whereas not all clinics necessarily do a full general examination, it is vital to the doctor to be able to examine the genitalia both externally and internally, because, for reasons that should be clear from preceding chapters, it is impossible to make an accurate diagnosis without such examination.

After external examination of the pubic region and vulva, the doctor will pass a speculum into the vagina and take the various samples that he needs from the vagina and cervix. After the vaginal examination a small sample will be taken from the urethra as this site may also be infected or may show signs of inflammation. In a few cases, it may be necessary to look at and take samples from the rectum. After these various tests have been taken, a bimanual examination of the pelvis is performed. If there are any spots or sores, then tests can be taken for Herpes simplex virus or for the treponeme of syphilis at the time of the genital examination, and likewise, genital warts can be treated with local applications of podophylline or acid.

In many clinics the genital examination is followed by a 'general' examination which may include feeling the breasts for lumps, a blood-pressure recording, and a look at the skin from the scalp to the soles of the feet. A sample of urine is usually needed either for simple testing in the clinic or to be sent off to the laboratory for more sophisticated tests. At the first visit it is usual to take a sample of blood after the examination proper is over.

After she has dressed, the female patient will be asked to wait while the various samples that have been taken for immediate microscopy are stained and examined. For a new patient this whole process may take upwards of an hour, after which she will see the doctor again and, if anything has been found, will be started on appropriate treatment. In perhaps 50 per cent of cases the final diagnosis depends on confirmatory results from the pathology laboratory and these take from two to seven days to come back to the clinic. If the tests are negative at the time of the initial examination, it is quite a good idea to ask the doctor whether he thinks there is likely to be any infection present or what he believes your symptoms are due to. The important thing to remember, however, is that in many cases no definitive diagnosis can be made until the results have come back from the laboratory and the fact that nothing has been found *at the time* of the first visit does not mean that the follow-up visit should be missed. Always return for the results of your tests!

A male attendance

After the initial booking-in, the man's progression through the clinic differs only in detail from the woman's. He must expect to be asked, like the woman, about his recent sexual encounters and whether a condom was used or not. Fellatio and cunnilingus are not regarded as perversions, rather as variations of normal sexual behaviour, and a punitive or disapproving approach from the doctor is a thing of the past. The same change in attitude is seen with regard to male homosexuals. Since the alteration of the law on homosexual acts between consenting adults, there has been a startling increase in the number of male patients who are prepared to talk freely about their homosexuality, and this can only be to the good, as they do appear to have a considerably higher chance of acquiring certain of the sexually transmitted conditions.

After the history has been taken, the doctor will want to examine the penis and, if relevant, the anus for signs of discharge, spots, or sores. Following this examination, urethral tests or proctoscopy may be performed, the latter if rectal intercourse has taken place. The commonest complaint in males is that of non-specific urethritis (NSU), and this can be diagnosed at the time of the first visit in the majority of cases. There is also a good chance of diagnosing gonorrhoea, if present, on this first occasion, unlike the case in women.

If syphilis is suspected, a 'dark-ground' or 'dark-field' examination may be performed on serum from a sore or rash. For this the sore is gently scraped and any fluid that exudes can then be looked at under the microscope. The sores are usually relatively painless, and this procedure, like the urethral investigation, need give no cause for alarm.

Following the genital tests and examination, there may be a general examination and a blood-test will be carried out. There will then be a wait while the various samples are examined under the microscope, and finally the results will be given by the doctor, and treatment prescribed as necessary. The male is lucky in that he is more likely to leave the clinic with a diagnosis at the end of his first visit.

Because urinating tends to wash out the urethra, and because the urethra can be such a rich source of diagnostic material, the doctors will always prefer a male patient to have held his urine, if possible, for three hours or more before attending for tests. If urine has been passed recently and there is therefore some doubt about the diagnosis, the patient may be asked to return for an early morning specimen (EMS) the next day. For this investigation the patient must attend the clinic in the early morning having held his urine all night.

In some clinics where the work-load is heavy, the actual tests from males may be taken by one of the technicians rather than the doctor. Most of the technicians are either members of the Institute of Technical Venereology, or trained nurses, or both.

Because of the potential seriousness of gonorrhoea or syphilis, if left untreated, nearly all the clinics in the United Kingdom have on their staff contact-tracers whose prime aim is to ensure that all efforts are made to persuade possible contacts of patients with either disease to attend for investigation. This may simply involve a talk with the infected patient explaining the way in which the diseases are transmitted and asking that he or she make every effort to persuade the contacts to attend. In some cases, however, the information on contacts may be slender, particularly if the sexual encounter followed a pick-up in a pub or resulted from a drunken all-night party which had been gate-crashed, and the contact-tracer may then be involved in trips, often abortive, to the Jolly Fig and Navel in the seedier part of town to try to locate Suzie – '... the one with the long blonde hair, pink mini-skirt, and acne'.

Finally, the staff of the clinic is completed by a social worker, whose role it is to try to sort out the non-medical problems that often go hand-in-hand with any infections. This may simply be a matter of explaining once again the implications of the diseases in terms of any personal relationships, giving advice about contraceptive clinics, or just lending a sympathetic ear while the patient unburdens his or her problems.

Special procedures

Blood-letting. Having blood taken, like many other minor medical procedures, is much worse in prospect than in practice. Blood is needed primarily to detect the presence of antibodies to the treponeme of syphilis, which may indicate either present or past infection. It is also useful for identifying the virus of type-B hepatitis. Although there are literally hundreds of blood-tests that can be performed in medical practice, it is usually only the serological tests for syphilis that are needed in the genito-urinary medicine clinic, and there is no point in asking, as many patients do, for their blood-group or their haemoglobin level, as these investigations will not have been done. Blood is taken, these days, with disposable (and therefore sharp) needles from a vein, usually in the arm. Veins can be identified by their faintly blue colour and they may be made to stand out by restricting the flow of blood back to the heart. Since the pressure of blood in the arteries is greater than that in the veins, an accumulation of blood occurs, making it easier to identify and puncture a vein. To this end a tourniquet of rubber tubing or other elastic material is usually placed around the upper arm. This tourniquet is released before the needle is withdrawn from the vein to prevent the back-pressure which has built up from causing the blood to spurt out and form a bruise.

Urethral tests. In order to ascertain the cause of a urethritis, it is necessary to obtain material from just inside the urethral meatus. Simply examining the purulent discharge does not give accurate enough answers. So the discharge itself is wiped away, and a small platinum loop or a cotton-wool-tipped orange stick is gently inserted into the urethral meatus, and samples from the urethra are plated out on the relevant culture media while others are smeared onto a microscope slide for staining and examination.

The two-glass test. This is a simple way for the doctor to assess urethritis. The male patient is asked to pass a little urine (perhaps the equivalent of two tablespoons) into one glass beaker and then to pass more into a second beaker. If there is a significant urethritis, this can be adduced by the presence of 'threads' or other solid material in the first glass. This first sample can be spun down and the solid matter can be stained and microscopically examined. Not all threads indicate urethritis, as collections of mucus and the secretions of the various glands can all produce 'bits' in the urine which may be mistaken for evidence of inflammation or infection if there is no microscopic examination. Often there are phosphates, a sort of salt, in the urine, which give it a cloudy appearance. Addition of acetic acid to the urine sample dissolves the salts and clears the urine.

Urethroscopy. This particular investigation is rarely performed nowadays but can still be useful in cases of treatment-resistant urethritis. A thin metal 'telescope', lubricated on the outside, is inserted into the urethra and by means of a light-source at its tip, the inside of the urethra can be examined for cysts, warts, herpetic ulcers, or infected urethral glands. It is possible to blow small amounts of air into the urethra by means of a balloon-valve, and in this way see if there are any strictures in the anterior urethra.

Vaginal examination. This is the most important part of the female examination. After inspection of the vulva and the skin surrounding the external genitalia, the doctor will pass a speculum into the vagina. The speculum is a metal or plastic device, which keeps the walls of the vagina (which are normally in close apposition) apart so that the cervix can be seen and samples can be taken accurately. To facilitate this examination, the woman lies on her back with her legs raised towards her chin and the knees or ankles supported. Although undeniably a somewhat indelicate position, it enables the examining doctor to get a good view of the vagina and cervix. The speculum, which is warmed before use, is smaller than an erect penis and does not normally produce any pain or discomfort when used. If there is a marked vaginitis, it may be necessary to use one of the smaller sizes of speculum but, even then, any discomfort should be minimal.

By performing this examination, the doctor is able to assess the nature and consistency of any vaginal discharge and take samples for microscopic and cultural analysis. Commonly he will be looking for evidence of thrush or trichomonal infection, but may also take samples for the other organisms that are found in the vagina from time to time. Following the vaginal tests, but at the same examination, tests are taken from the cervix. A cervical smear may be taken, which is specially stained in the laboratory (the Papanicolaou smear) and examined for evidence of early cancer of the cervix. Although this sounds as if it might be extremely uncomfortable, the cervix, like the vagina, is surprisingly poorly supplied with sensory nerve-endings, and a relaxed patient may be totally unaware that any samples are being taken from this site.

Bimanual examination. The doctor will often feel it necessary to examine the pelvic organs manually to assess whether there is evidence of pelvic inflammatory disease, fibroids in the uterus, or to see whether the uterus is enlarged when pregnancy is suspected. One or two fingers of one hand are inserted into the vagina, while the other hand feels the lower abdomen, and in this way, using both hands, the doctor can determine the outline, shape, and size of the contents of the pelvis. It is not a painful examination, but, as with all these tests, it is made considerably easier for both patient and doctor if the pelvic and abdominal muscles can be relaxed.

Proctoscopy. While it may seem obvious that the anus and rectum of a passive homosexual may be sites of infection and should therefore be examined, it may be difficult for women to understand why this same examination needs to be performed on them. Without dependence upon rectal intercourse having taken place, the gonococcus will be found in the rectum of 40 per cent of women who have gonorrhoea; and in 5 per cent it will be the only site to be involved by the infection. Gonorrhoea cannot be excluded in the female unless the rectum has been examined, and for this purpose a proctoscope, somewhat smaller than the vaginal speculum, is passed into the rectum so that samples can be taken for microscopy and culture. The proctoscope is lubricated, and, like the vaginal examination, this is not a painful procedure. Usually, proctoscopy is only performed on known gonorrhoea contacts and these make up only a small proportion of female patients seen in the clinic.

Prostatic massage. The prostate gland can be involved by infection, both gonococcal and non-gonococcal, and in order to tell whether it is inflamed it is helpful to be able to examine some of the fluid that it secretes. The prostate encircles the beginning of the urethra and is therefore rather difficult to get at directly. However, the back of the prostate is adjacent to the anterior wall of the rectum, and by gently massaging the gland from inside the rectum, a bead of fluid can be expressed and 'milked' along the urethra until it appears at the urethral meatus. It can then be examined and cultured like ordinary urethral samples.

Lumbar puncture. There is no procedure that strikes more fear and trepidation into the hearts of the ignorant and misinformed than the lumbar puncture. Often referred to as a 'lumbar punch', which sounds like a particularly nasty boxing foul, it is commonly thought to paralyse from the waist down those few lucky enough to survive the procedure, or at least render them impotent and incapable of sexual intercourse. All this is, of course, rubbish. The reason for performing lumbar puncture is to find out whether the central nervous system is involved by the syphilitic process in early or late syphilis. This is of importance since closer follow-up and longer treatment is needed in such cases. There are measurable changes in the cerebro-spinal fluid (the CSF) when neuro-syphilis is present, and therefore a sample of CSF needs to be obtained for analysis. The sample is collected via a small needle which is inserted into the space surrounding the spinal cord which is bathed by the CSF. The needle enters this space by passing between two of the lumbar vertebrae (the lowest of the bones that make up the spine) after the whole area has been infiltrated with local anaesthetic. Once the needle has entered the relevant space, several drops of CSF are collected into small bottles, which are sent to the laboratory for analysis. The needle is then withdrawn and the patient goes back to bed if he is an in-patient, or rests for two or three hours if an out-patient, before returning home to rest there. A small proportion of people develop a headache after lumbar puncture but this is usually because they have been too active too soon after the test.

Apart from the infiltration of the local anaesthetic, when the patient will feel a prick in the back, less painful than the anaesthetic for dental work, all that is felt is a pressure on the lower spine with occasionally a faint 'tingle' in one leg which simply signifies that the needle is in the right place. It doesn't cause paralysis! Because neurological syphilis is so rare these days, the call for lumbar puncture is limited. In one London clinic with thirty-five thousand patient visits in a year, only 30 lumbar punctures were performed, and so the prospect of this unreasonably unpopular test should not deter anyone from attending a clinic.

Urine tests. If it is thought that there may be infection in the bladder (cystitis) or kidneys, a special sample needs to be taken for laboratory analysis. This is the mid-stream urine (MSU) or clean-catch specimen of urine (CCSU). The idea is to let the initial sample of urine that is passed wash away any bacteria that are found around the urethral meatus or in the urethra, so that, if any bacteria are grown in the laboratory, it will be reasonably certain that they reflect infection actually inside the bladder or kidneys. After cleaning the external genitalia, a small amount of urine is passed and discarded. The area is again cleaned and the next sample of urine is collected in a sterile bottle and sent to the laboratory for analysis.

12

Control

There has been a world-wide increase in all the sexually transmitted diseases since the relative lull following the Second World War. Nobody knows exactly why this should have occurred, but one can identify several factors which play a part in furthering the survival of the many small organisms that have adapted to the sexual mode of transmission.

There are many different ways in which micro-organisms spread from person to person. Some depend on contagion – they need physical contact between an infected and a susceptible individual – while others are truly 'infectious', and, like the common cold, can be spread by infected droplets in the air, so that direct contact is not needed: it is enough to be in close proximity and to be breathing the same atmosphere. In some cases the faecal/oral route is used, and hands contaminated by faeces will transfer the infection to food, which is then eaten by others, or, as in the case of cholera, there may be faecal contamination of a water supply. Other organisms are happy to sit around waiting to be caught, like the bacteria responsible for tetanus, which can be found in fields, or the fungus responsible for athlete's foot, a ubiquitous inhabitant of the floors of swimming-pool changing rooms. Yet other organisms have become so specialized that they need an intermediate animal to act as host before they can become fully developed and infectious to man.

In this way all pathogenic organisms are dependent to a greater or lesser degree on external influences for their chance to spread and infect. The meningococcus is happiest when there is a crowded, closed community, such as a boarding school or an army camp, and it is in these sorts of institutions that epidemics of bacterial meningitis most often break out, rather than in rural communities where there is more space and air. Likewise, the malarial parasite has to depend on the presence of mosquitoes; and the various types of schistosome, which cause bilharzia in Africa, need a snail as an intermediate host before they can infect their definitive host, man.

The most important single factor common to all sexually transmitted organisms, that gives them a clear advantage over those responsible for

PLATE 7

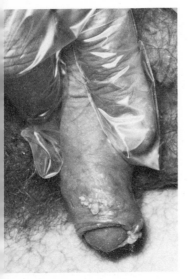

Penile warts

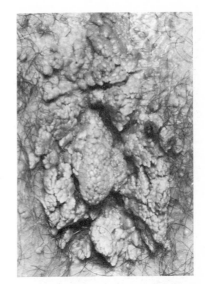

Perianal warts

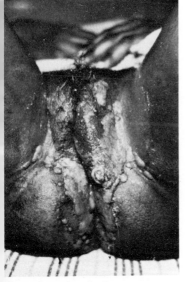

Granuloma inguinale

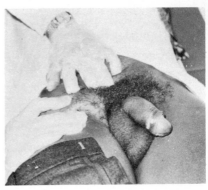

Chancroid with inguinal 'bubo'

PLATE 8

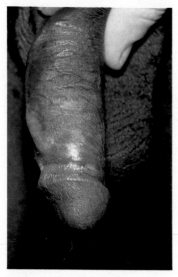

Herpes simplex infection of the penis

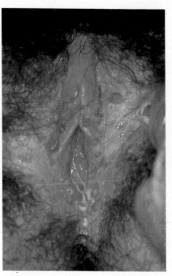

Herpes simplex infection of the vulva

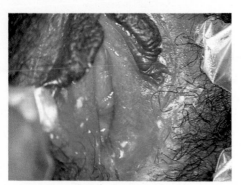

Candidal infection of the vulva

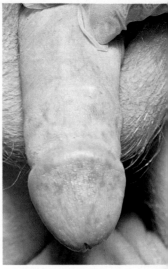

Candidal infection of the peni

many other infections, is that they are related to a world-wide and frequent activity during which there is close bodily contact, giving the optimum circumstances for transmission. They have attached themselves to the coat-tails of that strongest of all urges in the animal kingdom, bar that to survive, the sex drive.

The next clear advantage that these organisms possess is that, in general, they do not provoke a *useful* immunological response in the infected individual. Although one can observe and measure specific antibody increases in response to syphilis, gonorrhoea, herpes, or chlamydial infection, these antibodies are not strong enough to protect against further infection or, indeed, to eliminate the initial infection. This failure of the body to produce any adequate defence explains why, in spite of considerable expenditure of money and effort, there have been no successful vaccines produced against these diseases.

If a disease itself can stimulate immunity in the way, say, that smallpox does, then a programme of vaccination, health education, and vigorous contact-tracing can be expected to eliminate the infection entirely. This appears to have been the case with regards to smallpox, which, at the time of writing, seems to have been eradicated completely. By early 1979, there had been a fifteen-month period during which the only case of smallpox that had been reported from anywhere in the world occurred in Great Britain, and that originated in a virus research laboratory. In the case of sexually transmitted diseases, however, because natural infection does not produce immunity, producing a vaccine is particularly difficult, if not impossible.

The third factor favouring the spread of the sexually transmitted diseases is related to the signs and symptoms that they produce. In some cases there may be a genuine lack of symptoms, as is often the case in women, particularly with gonorrhoea; and in others the symptoms may not be directly referrable to the genitalia. If a man has had a 'silent' primary chancre, he will not immediately associate his secondary rash with syphilis, although he still is highly infectious. But probably more important than either lack of symptoms or misinterpretation of symptoms, is the stage in all these diseases when they are *presymptomatic*. There will inevitably be a period between catching an infection and the recognition of symptoms, be they discharge, dysuria, ulcer, or rash, when the patient will, nevertheless, be infectious, and unaware of it. It is reasonable to assume that only a small minority of people, those of a psychopathic bent, would have intercourse with someone when they knew that they, themselves, had a sexually transmitted infection, and yet these infections continue to be passed on.

The fourth factor, at present only of consequence with regard to the gonococcus, is the adaptation of the micro-organisms to therapy. We have seen that there has been a steady increase in the partial resistance of certain strains of gonococci to penicillin and, in the last few years, the emergence of some gonococci, the β-lactamase-producing ones, which are *totally* resistant to the antibiotic. A further result of the widespread use of antibiotics is the selection amongst a population of bacteria in favour of those strains that produce less symptoms. Reports from the United States of increasing numbers of *males* with gonorrhoea who are asymptomatic lends credence to this hypothesis. So far, there is no evidence of development of resistance by the treponeme to penicillin, either in the clinic or in the laboratory; nor have candida or chlamydia shown signs of resistance. Although resistance of *Trichomonas vaginalis* to metronidazole has been noted in the laboratory, it has not yet led to any problems with regard to treatment.

Social and educational factors

Ideas about the method of spread of sexually transmitted diseases have changed considerably in recent years and have some relevance to any attempts at controlling endemic levels of infection. The general belief in years gone by was that a 'pool' of infected women in the community was responsible for maintaining the level of infection. This pool was made up of prostitutes and ladies of easy virtue who infected their clients who then went on to infect their wives and girl-friends. This idea of a defined group acting as the source of infection implied that, were it only possible to identify them and isolate them from the rest of the population, it would be easy to eliminate the diseases from the community. This concept is inaccurate in two ways. Firstly, it is not so much the professional as the 'enthusiastic amateur' who passes on the diseases, and secondly, the spread of disease through the community is a dynamic rather than a static process. Instead of a defined sub-population that is almost continually infected and acts as a source of all other infection, it is more accurate and helpful to think of a 'wave' of infection passing through the community, occasionally, but by no means always, infecting the same people, but in general taking advantage of a high rate of partner-changing. Taking the wave analogy further, the crest of the wave represents those infections that have come to light, have been diagnosed, and treated, while the body of the wave and the trough preceding it, are the recently infected, asymptomatic or presymptomatic patients who have yet to emerge. These people will eventually become a 'crest' and be treated, but not before they themselves have passed the infection on to a further group. The distance between the waves could represent the incubation period and, taking the case of gonorrhoea, it is this which presents an insoluble problem in terms of control.

Assuming that the majority of men who have caught gonorrhoea will become symptomatic within a week or so, and will then take a few days to get treated, there is a limited time, perhaps ten days, during which they can pass on the infection. For the woman, the time-scale is of a different order. If a woman has caught gonorrhoea yet failed to develop any symptoms, she may have to rely on her next sexual partner developing gonorrhoea, having it diagnosed, and being able to trace her, before she becomes aware of her infection. Contact-tracing is designed to shorten this period, but it will almost always be longer for the female than the male, and the longer time interval makes it more likely that the infection will be passed on.

High-risk groups

Every time you go to bed with a new sexual partner, you put yourself at risk of acquiring a sexually transmitted infection, and, obviously, the more often partner-change occurs, the greater the risk becomes. When families are separated, the incidence of sexually transmitted disease amongst the menfolk rises and this is certainly seen in many countries of Europe where large immigrant work-forces make a contribution out of proportion to their numbers to the cases of sexually transmitted diseases. This is not because they bring disease with them, but because, deprived of their normal sexual outlets, they tend to have casual sexual relationships and to switch partners more often than would otherwise be the case.

The armed forces are for similar reasons more at risk than the civilian population, and this has been well known and occasionally condoned by their commanding officers. During the last war Montgomery was acutely aware of the problem and issued an order to his Division on the subject of prevention of venereal disease, after he had noted 44 cases in the twenty-eight days up to the 15th of November 1939. The order included a recommendation that it should be explained to soldiers wishing to purchase French letters that they should ask for a 'capote Anglaise'. Not that this was or is a peculiarly British problem. One unbelievable calculation during the Vietnam war maintained that, over a period of two years, nearly 50 per cent of GIs would have been infected with gonorrhoea.

In Great Britain, as elsewhere, it is the young who make up the majority of cases of sexually transmitted disease, and, perhaps as a reflection of their earlier sexual maturity, females under twenty are more often infected than males of the same age. In 1976, in England, there were 577 cases of gonorrhoea in the under-sixteens and 469 of these (81 per cent) were in females. Under twenty, the total number of cases was 12 044 of which 7308 were female. After that age the men rapidly caught up and overtook the women, so that the overall male to female ratio became 1·7 to 1. High-risk groups define themselves as including those people who have multiple sex partners, particularly if these are of a casual nature, and, of course, those whose *partners* are promiscuous.

Health education

The role of sex education in curbing the spread of sexually transmitted diseases is hard to assess. That young people should understand the mechanics of sex and reproduction is a received, if not a universally accepted, truth. It seems, however, to be difficult for educators to strike a balance of informing and yet not frightening their audience. Information about the sexually transmitted diseases may well have the effect of putting people off 'VD', but does not seem to have any effect on their sexual behaviour. Rather like a world war or drowning, it is something that happens to *other* people. Education of this sort, if badly done, can have the effect of scaring the pants off just those people one might be trying to persuade to remain fully clothed.

To rattle off a list of the horrendous diseases that can be sexually acquired to a group of sexually inexperienced schoolchildren is probably a highly ineffective method of reducing the incidence of infection, and serves merely as a weapon to instil fear and guilt. Exhortations to sexual continence, if they don't depend on religious or moral arguments, fall back on the threats of pregnancy or 'VD', and these have little relevance or meaning to young people who are sexually inexperienced. It might be better if the educators could acknowledge that sex is fun, and explain that most people find it so, and that youngsters embarking on sexual exploration are likely to be surprised by how strong their urges are. The problem was nicely summed up by a young girl quoted in the *Sunday Times* who said that, yes, she had had sex education but 'nobody explained to me how much I would want to do it'.

If it is accepted that many young people are going to have pre-marital sexual experience, some while still at school (and all the evidence suggests that this is exactly what is taking place) then it is better to concentrate on prophylaxis rather than scaremongering. Not only should the facts about contraception be made widely available to those who are likely to need it (and this can be done without it seeming that promiscuity is being advocated), but there should be information about where to go for contraceptive advice. The advantages of the barrier contraceptives, particularly the condom, should be *stressed*. The second point to be brought home is the risk attached to *rapid* partner changing – the fact that there will be a presymptomatic period when nothing wrong may be noticed yet sexually transmitted diseases can still be passed on. Thirdly, the open availability of clinics of genito-urinary medicine with the confidentiality that is attached to them and the fact that no letter of referral from the GP or school doctor is needed should be pointed out. The majority of clinic doctors are delighted to be consulted about worries and fears and would welcome the chance to educate, inform, and give advice.

Contraception

One of the reasons for the upsurge in sexually transmitted diseases since the mid-fifties is thought by many to be the change in contraceptive practice which has resulted from the widespread availability of the oral contraceptive. There is no doubt that the barrier contraceptives offer a great degree of protection against the acquisition or passing on of these diseases. The condom, or French letter, serves as a sound mechanical barrier not only to spermatazoa but also to bacteria and viruses. This fact has been well known for centuries and James Boswell, in his *London Journal* for 1763, describes his own use of the condom in various adventures with prostitutes in London, 'As I was coming home this night, I felt carnal inclinations raging through my frame. I determined to gratify them. I went to St James' Park, and, like Sir John Brute, picked up a whore. For the first time did I engage in armour, which I found but a dull satisfaction', and later, 'At night I strolled into the park and took the first whore I met, whom I without many words copulated with free from danger, being safely sheathed. She was ugly and lean and her breath smelt of spirits'. Although Boswell was in the habit of using his 'armour' with prostitutes, he felt safe to have intercourse with his new girl-friend, Louisa, without any protection and, when he contracted gonorrhoea from her, his physician told him 'that I had got an evident infection and that the woman who gave it me could not but know of it'. It is clear that Louisa had an *asymptomatic* gonococcal infection, but Boswell, unaware of this possibility, heaped odium and vituperation upon her, accusing her of deceit and baseness, corruption of body and mind, and having been rendered callous by a long course of disguised wickedness. One can't help feeling sorry for the poor woman, who had had no sexual relations with anyone for six months before she met Boswell and was clearly unaware that she had gonorrhoea.

For the condom to be effective as a prophylactive it is important that is should be used *throughout* intercourse and that there should be no contact between the genitalia before or after intercourse. The gonococcus can be regarded as having the same urge to infect as the sperm has to fertilize and, although no rhyme suggests itself immediately for the gonococcus, the message paraphrased in the sad tale of 'poor little Ermyntrude, who let one little sperm intrude' holds as well for sexually transmitted diseases as for pregnancy. The contraceptive cap used by the woman in combination with spermicidal cream or jelly has a similar, if slightly less effective, part to play in preventing transmission of infection.

In the days before the pill it was very much the man's role to look after contraception in casual sexual encounters, and a girl was unlikely to let him make love to her if he did not use a condom. These days many men don't give contraception a second thought, relying on the girl to tell them if she *isn't* on the pill.

The condom doesn't give complete protection, since infected secretions may be passed from person to person during the foreplay up to intercourse, and, of course, only the penis itself is protected, and scabies or crab-lice may be transferred even when the condom has been used correctly. If a syphilitic sore occurs at the base of the penis, it is known as a 'condom chancre'.

Prophylactic and epidemiological treatment

Both of these approaches to the problem of sexually transmitted diseases have been advocated singly and in combination and at first sight have some attractive points in their favour. Prophylactic treatment involves the taking of antibiotics just before or soon after intercourse in the hope of aborting any infection that might have been acquired. There are several drawbacks to this form of control, not least of which is the variety of medicaments that would need to be taken to cover all possible infections. Several antibiotics would need to be generally available and the promiscuous person might find themselves on more or less continuous treatment. Quite apart from the side-effects of many of these antibiotics, some of which are potentially very serious, there would be a general increase in the level of antibiotic resistance among a whole host of bacteria, with the result that many infections, at present comparatively easily dealt with, might end up virtually untreatable. The stringent laws against the indiscriminate use of antibiotics in farm animals came into being for exactly this reason, since it was found that, although the farm animals remained healthy, many of the bacteria that they carry which are pathogenic to man were becoming resistant.

Such prophylactic treatment for the venereal diseases was one of the features of the control policy by the Americans in South-East Asia, where, combined with epidemiological treatment, it resulted in many sexually active people having intercourse with sub-optimal levels of penicillin in their blood-streams, giving the gonococcus an unequalled opportunity to adapt to the antibiotic. If one had been given the problem of trying to make the gonococcus resistant to antibiotics in the 'field' rather than in the laboratory, one could not have devised a better way of doing it. Not only was the overall level of antibiotic resistance in Vietnam three or four times that found elsewhere in the world, but the evocatively named 'Vietnam Rose' emerged, which, while not being *totally* resistant like the β-lactamase-producing strains, needed a dose of penicillin so large that the average buttock simply wasn't big enough to accommodate it.

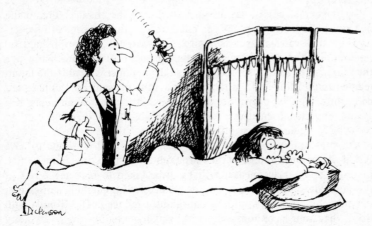

'This is going to hurt you more than your friend.'

Epidemiological treatment is another control measure advocated by the Americans, and this works on the principle that if a body has been in contact with someone known to be suffering from a venereal disease, then it is reasonable to treat them as if they themselves were suffering from the infection. The trouble with this approach is that it becomes apparent very soon that diagnostic tests are of secondary importance if the patient is going to be treated anyway, and this leads to all sorts of problems. What, for instance, do you do about the contacts of gonorrhoea contacts and what do you do about *their* contacts? Work from this country has shown that up to one third of female gonorrhoea contacts do not in fact have the disease, for one reason or another, and in one series from the States, only 30 per cent of such contacts could be shown to be harbouring the gonococcus. Some American authorities advocate a 'cluster' policy when dealing with syphilis or gonorrhoea. Having diagnosed a case of gonorrhoea, say, they try to pull in all the social acquaintances of the known case so that they may all be treated epidemiologically. 'All those who were at Saturday's all-night party on East 53rd Street please attend promptly for treatment'.

That these approaches are manifestly inefficient is borne out by the high rates of gonorrhoea and the high levels of resistance among the gonococci in the United States. A good indicator of how well a VD control programme is working is the prevalence of gonorrhoea in antenatal clinics. In the United Kingdom, less than one case in a hundred is picked up when pregnant mothers are randomly screened. In the USA the figure is nearer five cases in a hundred. There is little place for either prophylactic or epidemiological treatment in a well-run VD-control programme.

What general advice can be given to lessen the chances of catching one of the sexually transmitted diseases? The first, and most obvious, measure that can be taken is not to 'sleep around'. However, logic no more enters into sexual behaviour than it does into smoking, and while the majority of smokers would endorse the arguments against the habit, recognition of the risks attached does not, in general, modify their behaviour. Equally, only more so, with sex. In the heat of an impending sexual experience, matters such as the possibility of pregnancy or catching VD pale into insignificance.

On the assumption, then, that many people will continue to have casual sexual encounters, as they probably have since time immemorial, there are still certain measures that can be taken to reduce the risk. If the male always used a condom, the chances of his catching a disease or infecting his partner would be enormously reduced. The trouble with this is that using a condom is thought by many to reduce the spontaneity of the act and also to lessen the sensitivity and the sexual pleasure: 'like making love in gum-boots'. This is, of course, an exaggeration, but the fact remains that a lot of young people have strong, if ill-founded, objections to using a protective. This is where the female can have a strong influence. She may insist that her boyfriend uses a condom and, just as young men used to carry them around 'just in case', so she could have a supply in her handbag and if she says that she has just come off the pill and might get pregnant, she will probably be able to persuade her partner to use one. No condom, no sex.

It is also important that the risks of *frequent* partner switching should be recognized. It is not just that there is obviously more chance of catching something the more sexual experiences you have, but that there should be a 'reasonable' time interval between partners. By this is meant a period long enough for there to be a chance for symptoms or signs of infection to develop. This is more true of the male, who is more likely to notice something wrong than the female. If all those people who had no steady relationship would wait at least six weeks between sexual experiences with different partners, the problems associated with sexually transmitted diseases would, if not vanish overnight, suddenly become much easier to control. It would also help if people more often knew the names and addresses of those they went to bed with on a casual basis.

Another piece of sound, if impractical, advice to the female is to examine her new partner before intercourse takes place. One best-selling sex manual blithely suggests that this examination can form part of the sexual foreplay. This is all very well for the old-time professional prostitute who, if she knows her trade at all, will first perform a minute 'short arm inspection' and then unroll a condom over the erect penis, but for someone stuck in the parlour with the lights off, or groping in the back seat of a clapped-out Ford, it doesn't even enter into the realms of wishful thinking.

Washing the genitalia and passing urine after intercourse have always been advocated as ways of reducing the chances of catching an infection, but the likelihood of these measures being effective is small. What is more probable is that scrubbing and bathing the affected parts in strong household antiseptics, a popular prophylactic procedure, will lead to traumatic or chemical injury.

Once someone has put him or herself at risk, it is important to keep an eye open for the development of symptoms, and if in any doubt at all to go to a clinic for a check-up. A large proportion of patients attending the clinics up and down the country attend to be reassured that they have no disease rather than because they know themselves to be infected, and all clinics are happy to perform such checks. Do not expect, however, to be given the all-clear if you come for a check the day after you've been at risk. Many of the diseases, although they can be passed on soon after they have been acquired, take a few days before they can be diagnosed or excluded. Finally, if one of the less important, 'minor' sexually transmitted diseases such as crabs, molluscum, or scabies develops, it is always worth while making sure that there are no other, more important infections as well.

Glossary

abscess: A walled-in collection of pus.

acute: Early (in the course of a disease), relatively severe, sharp; opposite of chronic.

aneurysm: A dilatation in the wall of an artery.

anterior: In front of.

antibiotic: A chemical substance, often derived originally from a micro-organism, capable of killing or preventing the growth or division of bacteria.

antibody: A protein elaborated by the body's defence mechanisms which neutralizes specific 'foreign' substances, such as bacteria, viruses, or other proteins.

antigen: Any substance which, when introduced into the body, is capable of stimulating the formation of antibodies.

aorta: The largest artery, which supplies all the other large arteries. Syphilis may attack this vessel with resulting 'aortitis' and aneurysm formation.

arthritis: Inflammation of one or more joints. This may complicate gonorrhoea, non-specific infection, or syphilis

Australia antigen: The virus responsible for type-B (serum) hepatitis.

axilla: The armpit.

bacterium: Microscopic one-celled organism. Gonorrhoea, syphilis, chancroid, non-specific infection, LGV, and granuloma inguinale are bacterial infections, Bacteria are usually amenable to treatment with antibiotics, although the sensitivity of given bacteria to different drugs may vary considerably.

balanitis: Inflammation of the glans penis.

balano-posthitis: Inflammation of the foreskin and glans penis.

Bartholin's gland: A paired gland situated at the lower third of the labium majus which secretes a thin mucus to aid lubrication during sexual intercourse.

bejel: One of the tropical treponematoses.

biopsy: The removal of a piece of tissue for examination in the laboratory

bubo: The swelling caused by infection and inflammation in a lymphatic gland, particularly in the groin or axilla.

bullous: A skin lesion like a large blister.

Glossary of terms

Candida albicans: A yeast-like fungus responsible for thrush, vaginal discharge, and balanitis.

cardiovascular: Referring to the heart and blood-vessels.

carrier: Someone infected by a micro-organism, but who shows no sign of the infection, while remaining infectious to others.

cerebro-spinal fluid (CSF): The fluid bathing the brain and spinal cord.

cervix: Literally a neck; in this context refers to the neck of the womb. Inflammation of the cervix is called cervicitis. The site most commonly infected by the gonococcus is the inside of the cervix, the endocervix.

chancre: The sore or ulcer manifesting the primary stage of syphilis.

chancroid: A tropical sexually transmitted disease caused by *Haemophilus ducreyi.*

chronic: Long-standing; the opposite of acute.

clitoris: A sensitive, erectile organ, analogue of the male penis.

coccus: A round bacterium. The organism causing gonorrhoea is a coccus.

commensal: A micro-organism that lives in or on a body without causing disease.

condylomata acuminata: Venereal warts. Caused by a virus, they should not be confused with:

condylomata lata: The wart-like growths found around the anus and genitalia in secondary syphilis. They are highly infectious.

congenital: Present at birth, having been acquired *in utero*.

conjunctivitis: Inflammation or infection of the lining of the eyelid and the covering of the eye.

crabs: Infestation with pubic lice.

culture: The process of growing micro-organisms in the laboratory to help their identification.

cutaneous: Referring to the skin.

cyst: A sac, often containing fluid.

cystitis: Infection or inflammation of the bladder.

dermatitis: An inflammation of the skin.

disseminated gonococcal infection (DGI): The illness that follows, spread (usually via the blood-stream) to other parts of the body.

discharge: An excretion of fluid, usually from the vagina or urethra.

dysentery: Infection of the bowel by certain defined mircro-organisms. Reiter's syndrome may occasionally follow dysentery.

dysmenorrhoea: Pain at the time of the menstrual period.

dyspareunia: Pain felt by the woman at sexual intercourse. It may be superficial, as in herpetic infection of the vulva, or deep, as in salpingitis.

dysuria: Pain or discomfort associated with passing urine.

ectopic: In the wrong place. In an ectopic pregnancy the fertilized ovum implants outside the uterus, often in the fallopian tube. This is more likely to occur if there is a past history of salpingitis.

elephantiasis: Enlargement of the skin and tissues following blockage of lymphatic drainage channels. May occur in LGV.

endocarditis: Inflammation or infection of the lining of the heart and its valves. Follows rheumatic fever and, very rarely, disseminated gonococcal infection.

endometrium: The blood-rich lining of the uterus. If pregnancy does not occur this lining is shed each month and constitutes the menstrual flow.

endemic: A steady state of infection in a community varying little year by year.

enzyme: A biologically active protein facilitating biochemical reactions.

epidemic: A sudden large increase in the level of an infection in a community.

epidemiology: The study of patterns of disease. Epidemiological treatment means the treatment, on suspicion, before or without diagnosis of the disease.

epididymis: The coiled first part of the tube connecting the testis to the urethra. Infection gives rise to epididymitis or, if the testis is involved as well, epididymo-orchitis.

epithelium: The layer of cells covering or lining other tissue. Skin and mucous membranes are epithelia.

erosion: Literally an 'eating-away' or ulcer, it refers specially to a benign and common condition affecting the cervix in which the normal epithelium on its vaginal portion is replaced by epithelium from the endocervix. It is an unimportant variation on the normal.

exudate: A fluid 'oozed out' like sweat. The result of inflammation, often containing many white cells. The urethral discharge in gonorrhoea is an exudate.

fallopian tubes: These connect the ovaries and the uterus. Infection in the tubes is called salpingitis.

fellatio: Oral stimulation of the penis.

fistula: A canal or track connecting an internal organ with another or with the outside world. Usually the result of disease.

Frei tests: A skin test used in the diagnosis of LGV. Rarely performed because of shortage of antigen.

frequency (of micturition): Passing urine more often than usual. It may be diurnal, nocturnal, or both. It is more often a symptom of cystitis than of sexually transmitted disease.

FTA-Abs test: short for the fluorescent treponemal antibody absorbed test, the FTA is the most reliable specific blood-test for treponemal disease.

fungi: These are vegetable organisms of a low order of development. Although mushrooms, toadstools, and moulds are more familiar, there are several fungi pathogenic to man. *Candida albicans* is the most ubiquitous of these.

Glossary of terms

genito-urinary: Referring to the reproductive and excretory systems. The latter with reference to the kidneys, bladder, etc.

gland: An organ that secretes a substance. The term is loosely used to describe the lymph nodes which are found throughout the body. 'Swollen glands' implies infection.

gonococcus: *Neisseria gonorrhoeae*, the bacterium responsible for gonorrhoea. It is a gram-negative coccus.

gonorrhoea: The commonest of the 'true' venereal diseases. Characterized by dysuria and urethral discharge in men and few symptoms in women.

gram-stain: A method of staining micro-organisms to facilitate their microscopic examination and identification.

granuloma inguinale: A tropical or sub-tropical sexually transmitted disease caused by *Donovania granulomatis*.

gumma: The inflammatory tumour or infiltration found in tertiary syphilis.

Herpes simplex: The virus responsible for 'cold sores'. Type I is usually responsible for infection of the mouth and lips, while type II more often affects the genitalia.

Hutchinson's triad: Three stigmata of congenital syphilis: Hutchinson's teeth, nerve deafness, and interstitial keratitis, a clouding of the front of the eye.

hypertrophy: An increase in the size of an organ or tissue.

Jarisch–Herxheimer reaction: A reaction that follows the start of treatment for syphilis perhaps caused by the break-up of the bacteria responsible. There is a brief flu-like illness and syphilitic lesions may get temporarily worse.

incidence: The number of cases occurring in a defined area during a specified period of time.

incubation period: The time between acquiring an infection and developing signs or symptoms.

indurated: Hard.

infectivity: The likelihood of a given infection being passed on to those exposed to it. Very few infections have an infectivity of 100 per cent. The infectivity of most sexually transmitted diseases is unknown.

inflammation: The reaction of tissues to injury or infection. Inflammation is characterized by pain, swelling, redness, and warmth. White cells are attracted to areas of inflammation.

inguinal: Referring to the groin region.

intracellular: Literally 'inside a cell'. A requirement for the diagnosis of gonorrhoea under the microscope.

introitus: The entrance to the vagina.

in vitro: Referring to the results of tests or experiments in the laboratory in test-tubes or other apparatus, in contrast to:

in vivo: which refers to the effects of such tests in living animals or humans.

iritis: Inflammation of the iris of the eye.

labia: The lips around the vagina. Labia minora are the small lips surrounding the introitus, and outside these are the larger labia majora.

labial: Confusingly, usually refers to the lips around the mouth. Thus labial herpes is an infection on the face rather than the genitalia.

latent: Hidden or concealed. Often refers to the presence of a disease which doesn't show itself.

lateral: At the side, or to the side of.

lesion: A local wound or disruption of tissue. The result of a pathological process or trauma.

leucocyte: A white blood-cell.

lues: An old-fashioned word for syphilis.

lymphadenopathy: A swelling of the lymph nodes.

lymphocyte: A sort of white cell formed in the lymph glands, concerned with immunity and antibody production.

lymphogranuloma venereum (LGV): A tropical or sub-tropical sexually transmitted disease caused by *Chlamydia trachomatis*.

lumbar puncture: A procedure in which the cerebro-spinal fluid is sampled to ascertain whether infection is involving the central nervous system.

macule: A discoloured spot on the skin, not raised above the normal surface. A macule may evolve into a papule, vesicle, or pustule.

medium: The substance on which micro-organisms may be cultured in the laboratory.

meningitis: Inflammation (usually infection) of the meninges, which are the layers surrounding the brain and spinal cord. Meningitis occurs in secondary syphilis and rarely in gonorrhoea.

menstruation: The monthly loss from the uterus.

metronidazole: A drug useful against *Trichomonas vaginalis* and certain anaerobic bacteria (those that do not like oxygen).

micturition: Passing urine.

mucous membrane: The shiny epithelium lining the cavities of the body open to the air, such as the mouth, respiratory tract, and genitalia.

neonatal: Referring to the period soon after birth.

neoplasm: A tumour or new growth.

neurosyphilis: The involvement of the nervous system by syphilis. The best known manifestations are tabes dorsalis and general paralysis of the insane (GPI).

nodule: Small palpable swelling, usually in the skin.

non-specific urethritis (NSU): Also known as non-gonococcal urethritis (NGU), this is the most common form of urethritis.

Glossary of terms

oedema: Swelling due to retention of fluid.

ophthalmia neonatorum: Infection of the eye of the newborn baby. The gonococcus used to be the most common cause, more recently chlamydia has been implicated in many cases.

orchitis: Inflammation or infection of the testis.

ovary: The paired female sex gland which produces the ovum and also makes sex hormones.

palpable: Discernible by touch.

pandemic: A disease that has spread all over the world.

papule: A skin lesion raised above the surface.

parasite: A plant or animal that lives on or within another organism at the expense of that organism.

pathogen: A micro-organism capable of producing disease.

pelvic inflammatory disease (PID): Infection of the pelvic organs in the female, often used synonymously with salpingitis.

penicillin: The first antibiotic. Still the first line of treatment for gonorrhoea and syphilis.

peritonitis: Infection involving the lining of the abdominal organs, the peritoneum. Often associated with acute appendicitis, it may complicate salpingitis if this is not treated early.

pH: A measure of the acidity of a fluid. The lower the pH, the more acid.

pharynx: The throat.

phimosis: A constriction of the foreskin preventing it from being drawn back over the penis. Occasionally, having been retracted, the foreskin cannot be brought forward again. This is called paraphimosis. Both these conditions are sometimes brought on as a result of sexually transmitted disease.

pinta: A tropical treponemal disease caused by *Treponema careatum*. Not sexually transmitted.

placenta (afterbirth): The organ separating the maternal from the foetal circulation in the uterus, while allowing the transfer of nutrients and oxygen and the elimination of waste material.

polymorphonuclear leucocyte: The white blood-cell that is responsible for the formation of pus, hence its common name, the 'pus' cell. It is phagocytic, that is it can ingest bacteria and other debris.

posterior: Behind, at the back of.

prevalence: The number of cases of a disease in an area at a given point in time.

proctitis: Inflammation or infection of the rectum. Common among male homosexuals, it may be caused by the gonococcus or may be a manifestation of non-gonococcal infection.

prostatitis: Inflammation or infection of the prostate gland.

protozoon: A large single-celled organism. *Trichomonas vaginalis* is a protozoon.

pruritus: Itchiness or irritation.

purulent: Made up of pus.

124

Glossary of terms

pustule: A raised spot on the skin containing pus.

reagin: A group of antibodies which increase in quantity when there is active syphilis. It is reagin that is measured by the non-specific blood-tests such as the WR or the VDRL.

Reiter's disease: A condition that occasionally follows non-specific urethritis and bacillary dysentery. Typically there is a urethritis, arthritis, conjunctivitis, and skin lesions.

rhagades: Small linear scars around the corners of the mouth seen in some patients with congenital syphilis.

rod: A long bacterium. The causative organism of chancroid is a rod.

salpingitis: Infection of the fallopian tubes. Gonorrhoea used to be the most common cause but is now isolated in well under 50 per cent of cases.

scabies (the itch): A contagious skin disease caused by a mite, *Sarcoptes scabiei.*

seminal vesicle: A small secretory sac attached to the vas deferens.

septicaemia: The presence of bacterial toxins in the blood.

serological tests for syphilis (STS): The blood-tests used to diagnose syphilis. They include the reagin tests as well as the specific tests.

serum: The portion of blood left after the solid components have been removed. Also describes the exudate from a chancre, which can be examined microscopically.

sinus: A hollow space or channel usually caused by a pathological process.

slide: The glass microscope slide on which material from potentially infected sites is placed prior to staining and examination.

snuffles: The heavy watery discharge from the nose and pharynx of the new-born child with congenital syphilis. The exudate is teeming with treponemes.

spirochaete: A member of the genus to which *Treponema pallidum* belongs.

stat: To be given at once (of medicines).

stricture: An abnormal narrowing in a tube or channel. Urethral stricture is one of the late complications of untreated gonorrhoea in the male.

suppuration: The formation of pus, usually leading to its discharge as from an abcess.

syphilis: One of the oldest of the venereal diseases, caused by *Treponema pallidum.*

systemic: Not localized, involving the whole of the body.

testis: The paired male sex gland, which produces spermatazoa and the male sex hormones.

tetracycline: Like penicillin, an antibiotic, but one that is active against a wider variety of bacteria. The most useful treatment for NSU.

thrombosis: The development of a clot or thrombus in a blood vessel.

Glossary of terms

titre: The measure of the amount of antibody present in the blood by a method of dilution.

TPHA and TPI: Two specific blood-tests for the detection of syphylis.

trauma: A wound or injury, not necessarily of a severe nature.

treponema pallidum: The causative organism of syphilis.

trichomonas vaginalis: The protozoon responsible for a vaginal infection in women and a low-grade urethritis in men.

urethra: The tube connecting the bladder with the outside world.

urethritis: inflammation or infection in the urethra.

urgency: The feeling of need to pass water immediately.

uterus: The womb. The organ in which the foetus develops.

vagina: The channel into which the erect penis is inserted during sexual intercourse.

vaginitis: Inflammation of the vagina. Most often due to *Candida albicans*, although other organisms, particularly trichomonas, may be responsible.

vas deferens: The tube connecting the testis to the urethra.

virus: The smallest of the micro-organisms to affect man. They are not susceptible to antibiotics.

venereal: Having to do with sex. From Venus, the goddess of love.

VDRL: The Venereal Disease Reference Laboratory blood-test, one of the easiest and cheapest of the non-specific blood-tests for syphilis.

vesicle: A small blister. Characteristic of herpetic infection at an early stage.

vulva: The female external genital area.

vulvovaginitis: Inflammation of the vulva and vagina together.

warts: Transmissible skin growths caused by viruses.

Wasserman Reaction (WR): The first blood-test used for the diagnosis of syphilis in the first decade of this century. Now superseded by more modern tests.

yaws: A treponemal disease of tropical climes caused by *Treponema pertenue*. It is not sexually transmitted.

List of clinics

England

STD clinics in the provinces

County and town	Address and telephone number of clinic	
	Avon	
Bath	Royal United Hospital, Combe Park, Bath.	Bath 28331 ext. 444 and 423
Bristol	Bristol Royal Infirmary, Upper Maudlin Street, Bristol.	Bristol 290431/2/3/4
Weston-super-Mare	Weston-super-Mare General Hospital, The Boulevard, Weston-super-Mare.	Weston-super-Mare 25211
	Bedfordshire	
Bedford	Bedford General Hospital, Kempton Road, Bedford.	Bedford (0234) 55155
Luton	St. Mary's Hospital, 11A Dunstable Road, Luton.	Luton 21261/414243
	Berkshire	
Reading	Royal Berkshire Hospital, Reading.	Reading 85111, ext. 299
Windsor	King Edward VII Hospital, Windsor.	Windsor 60441
	Buckinghamshire	
Aylesbury	Royal Bucks Hospital, Aylesbury.	Aylesbury 4411
High Wycombe	Wycombe General Hospital, High Wycombe.	High Wycombe 26161
Wolverton	Wolverton Health Centre/Day Hospital, Gloucester Road, Wolverton, Milton Keynes.	0908 316633
	Cambridgeshire	
Cambridge	Addenbrookes Hospital, Hills Road, Cambridge.	Cambridge 45151, ext. 7239
Peterborough	Peterborough District Hospital.	Peterborough 67451

List of clinics

Cheshire

Chester	Chester Royal Infirmary, St. Martins's Way, Chester.	Chester 28261, ext. 321
Crewe	Special Clinic, 8 Herdman Street, Crewe.	0270 2019
Warrington	Warrington General Hospital, Lovely Lane, Warrington.	0925 35911

Cleveland

Middlesborough	Middlesborough General Hospital, Middlesborough.	0642 83133
Stockton-on-Tees	North Tees General Hospital, Stockton-on-Tees.	Stockton-on-Tees (0642) 62122
West Hartlepool	Hartlepool General Hospital, Hartlepool.	0429 66654 ext. 424

Cornwall

Falmouth	Falmouth Hospital, Falmouth.	0326 311841
Newquay	Newquay Hospital, Newquay.	063–73 3883
Penzance	West Cornwall Hospital, Penzance.	0736 2382, ext. 200
St. Austell	St. Austell Hospital, Edgcombe Road, St. Austell.	0726 2401
Truro	Royal Cornwall Hospital (City), Truro.	0872 3081

Cumbria

Barrow-in-Furness	Devonshire Road Hospital, Barrow-in-Furness.	0229 22760
Carlisle	Cumberland Infirmary, Carlisle.	0228 23444, ext. 544
Kendal	Westmorland County Hospital, Kendal.	0539 22641
Whitehaven	West Cumberland Hospital, Hensingham, Whitehaven.	0946 3181, ext. 441
Workington	Workington Infirmary.	0900 2244, ext. 253

Derbyshire

Chesterfield	Royal Hospital, Chesterfield.	Chesterfield 77271, ext. 217
Derby	Derbyshire Royal Infirmary, Derby.	Derby 47141, ext. 504

Devon

Barnstaple	North Devon Infirmary, Barnstaple.	Barnstaple 2291 ext. 025
Exeter	Royal Devon and Exeter Hospital, Barrack Road, Wonford, Exeter.	Anwering service: 34488; Exeter 77833, ext. 2422 (clinic)
Plymouth	Diagnostic and Treatment Centre, Plymouth General Hospital, Freedom Fields, Plymouth.	Plymouth 63609

List of clinics

| Torquay | Special Clinic, Torbay Hospital, Newton Road, Torquay. | Torquay 64567 |

Dorset

Bournemouth	Victoria Hospital, Gloucester Road, Boscombe.	Bournemouth 38548, ext. 1
Dorchester	Dorchester County Hospital, Dorchester.	Dorchester 3123, ext. 330
Weymouth	Portwey Hospital, Wyke Road, Weymouth.	Weymouth 4881, ext. 7

Durham

| Darlington | Darlington Memorial Hospital, Hundens Lane, Darlington. | Darlington 60100, ext. 45 |

Essex

Chelmsford	Chelmsford and Essex Hospital, New Writtle Street, Chelmsford.	Chelmsford 53481, ext. 27
Colchester	Essex County Hospital, Lexdon Road, Colchester.	Colchester 77341, ext. 459
Grays	Orsett Hospital, Grays Thurrock.	0375 5100, ext. 387
Romford	The Annexe, Old Church Hospital, Waterloo Road, Romford.	(70) 46090, ext. 3258/ 3259
Southend-on-sea	General Hospital, Prittlewell Chase, Southend-on-sea.	0702 48911, ext. 463/467

Gloucestershire

| Cheltenham | Cheltenham General Hospital, Sandford Road, Cheltenham. | Cheltenham 21344, ext. 278 |
| Gloucester | Gloucester Royal Hospital, Great Western Road, Gloucester. | Gloucester 21021, ext. 41 |

Greater Manchester

Ashton-under-Lyne	General Hospital, Darnton Road, Ashton-under-Lyne.	061 330 4321
Bolton	Public Health Department, Civic Centre, Bolton.	Bolton 22311, ext. 307/8; night: Bolton 23465
Bury	General Hospital, Walmersley Road, Bury.	061 764 2444, ext. 273
Manchester	St. Luke's Clinic, 1 Duke Street, Manchester. M3 4NJ	061 834 0585/ 834 0093
Manchester	Royal Infirmary, Oxford Road, Manchester. M13 9WL	061 273 3300, ext. 123
Oldham	Oldham and District General Hospital, Rochdale Road, Oldham	061 624 0420, ext. 121
Rochdale	Sparthfield Clinics, Manchester Road, Rochdale.	Rochdale 48827
Salford	Hope Hospital, Eccles Old Road, Salford. M6 8HD	061 789 5252, ext. 50
Stockport	St. Thomas' Hospital, Stockport.	061 480 7645

List of clinics

Wigan	Royal Albert Edward Infirmary, Wigan.	Wigan 44000, ext. 224

Hampshire

Basingstoke	Basingstoke District Hospital, Park Prewitt, Basingstoke.	0256 3202, ext. 6179; or 0256 52333
Portsmouth	St. Mary's General Hospital, Portsmouth.	Portsmouth 816941; or 22331 ext. 232
Southampton	44 Bullar Street, Southampton.	Southampton 34288, ext. 437/438
Winchester	Royal Hampshire County Hospital, Winchester.	Winchester 63535, ext. 154

Hereford and Worcester

Hereford	County Hospital, Hereford.	0432 68161, ext. 328
Worcester	Worcester Royal Infirmary, Castle Street, Worcester.	0905 27122, ext. 14

Hertfordshire

Bishops's Stortford	Herts and Essex Hospital, Bishop's Stortford.	0279 55191, ext. 61
St. Albans	St. Albans City Hospital, Normandy Road, St. Albans.	St. Albans 52211, ext. 228
Stevenage	New Lister Hospital, Stevenage.	0438 4333, ext. 578
Watford	Watford General Hospital, Vicarage Road, Watford.	Watford 44366, ext. 206

Humberside

Grimsby	Scartho Road Hospital, Grimsby.	South Humberside, 0472 79281 ext. 296; or 0472 70499
Hull	Mill Street Clinic, Kingston-on-Hull, North Humberside.	0482 2256 ext. 16
Scunthorpe	Scunthorpe General Hospital, Cliff Gardens, Scunthorpe.	South Humberside 0724 3481, ext. 451

Isle of Wight

Newport	St. Mary's Hospital, Newport.	Newport 4081, ext. 359

Kent

Canterbury	Kent and Canterbury Hospital, Canterbury.	Canterbury 52222
Dartford	West Hill Hospital, Dartford.	Dartford 23223, ext. 116
Folkestone	Old Harvey Grammer School, Foord Road, Folkestone.	Folkestone 58286
Gravesend	22 Cobham Street, Gravesend.	Gravesend 3061
Maidstone	West Kent General Hospital, Maidstone.	Maidstone 65411, ext. 260
Margate	Royal Seabathing Hospital, Canterbury Road, Margate.	Thanet 27903

130

List of clinics

Rochester	36 New Road, Rochester.	Medway 43343
Sheerness	Sheppey General Hospital, Minster.	Sheerness 2116, ext. 42
Tunbridge Wells	Kent and Sussex Hospital, Mount Ephraim, Tunbridge Wells.	0892 26111, ext. 107

Lancashire

Blackburn	Royal Infirmary, Blackburn.	Blackburn 55222, ext. 236 (day); 235 (night)
Blackpool	Municipal Health Centre, 156 Whitegate Drive, Blackpool.	Blackpool (0253) 63626
Burnley	General Hospital, Casterton Av., Burnley.	Burnley 25071, ext. 304/5 (day); 401 (night)
Lancaster	Royal Lancaster Infirmary, Lancaster.	Lancaster 65944, ext. 90
Preston	Preston Royal Infirmary, Preston.	Preston 54747, ext. 252

Leicestershire

Leicester	Leicester Royal Infirmary.	Leicester 541414, ext. 497/590
Loughborough	Loughborough Hospital.	0509 21 4867, ext. 23

Lincolnshire

Boston	Pilgrim Hospital, Boston.	Boston 4801, ext. 458
Grantham	Grantham and Kesteven General Hospital, Grantham.	0476 5232, ext. 213
Lincoln	Lincoln County Hospital.	0522 29921 ext. 378
Skegness	Skegness and District Hospital, Dorothy Avenue, Skegness.	0754 2401/2

Merseyside

Birkenhead	St. James' Hospital, Birkenhead.	(051) 652 3574, ext. 57
Liverpool	Newsham General Hospital, Liverpool.	(051) 263 7381, ext. 127
	Liverpool Royal Infirmary, Pembroke Place, Liverpool.	(051) 709 5511, ext. 210/253
	Seamen's Dispensary, Cleveland Square, Paradise Street, L'pool.	(051) 709 2165
St. Helens	Health Department Dispensary, 5 Parade Street, St. Helens.	St. Helens 24061, ext. 2303; or 22730
Southport	Southport General Infirmary, Pilkington Road, Southport.	Southport 42901, ext. 398

Norfolk

Great Yarmouth	Estcourt Hospital, Great Yarmouth.	Great Yarmouth 56222, ext. 346
Norwich	Norfolk and Norwich Hospital, Norwich.	Norwich 28377, ext. 3321
Kings Lynn	Kings Lynn General Hospital.	(0553) 61281, ext. 254

List of clinics

Northamptonshire

Kettering	Kettering General Hospital.	Kettering 81141, ext. 365
Northampton	Northampton General Hospital.	Northampton 34700, ext. 63; or 37203

Nottinghamshire

Mansfield	Mansfield and District General Hospital, West Hill Drive, Mansfield.	Mansfield 22414, ext. 442
Nottingham	General Hospital, Nottingham (Postern Street)	Nottingham 45989/45980
	City Hospital, Nottingham.	Nottingham 45989/45980

Oxfordshire

Oxford	Radcliffe Infirmary Oxford.	Oxford 46036

Salop

Shrewsbury	Clinic 9, Shrewsbury Hospital.	0743 52244

Somerset

Bridgwater	General Hospital, Bridgwater.	Bridgwater 51501, ext. 54
Taunton	East Reach Hospital, Taunton.	Taunton 3444, ext. 5054
Yeovil	District Hospital, Yeovil.	Yeovil 3870, ext. 382

Staffordshire

Burton-on-Trent	District Hospital Burton.	0283 66333, ext. 92
Stafford	General Infirmary, Stafford.	Stafford 58251, ext. 72
Stoke-on-Trent	Wellesley Street Centre, Stoke-on-Trent.	Stoke-on-Trent 22051
	O.P.D., Hartshill, Stoke-on-Trent.	Stoke-on-Trent 44161, ext. 4205

Suffolk

Bury St. Edmonds	West Suffolk District Hospital, Bury St. Edmonds.	Bury St. Edmonds 63131
Ipswich	Clinic 8, The Ipswich Hospital.	Ipswich 711011
Lowestoft	Lowestoft and North Suffolk Hospital, Lowestoft.	Lowestoft 65151, ext. 16

Surrey

Camberley	Frimley Park Hospital, Frimley.	Camberley 62121, ext. 4220
Guildford	Royal Surrey County Hospital, Guildford.	0483 73852
Redhill	East Surrey Hospital, Redhill.	Redhill 65081, ext. 11
Woking	Victoria Hospital, Woking.	Woking 5911, ext. 38

Sussex–East

Brighton	Royal Sussex County Hospital, Brighton.	Brighton 66611, ext. 39

List of clinics

Eastbourne	Avenue House, The Avenue, Eastbourne.	Eastbourne 37121, ext. 53
Hastings	Ore Hospital, Hastings. Royal East Sussex Hospital, Cambridge Road, Hastings.	0424 420801 0424 434513

Sussex–West

Chichester	Royal West Sussex Hospital, Broyle Road, Chichester.	Chichester 88122, ext. 781
Worthing	Worthing Hospital.	Worthing 205111, ext. 97

Tyne and Wear

Newcastle-on-Tyne	Ward 34, Newcastle General Hospital.	Newcastle 33320 and 35516
North Shields	Ward 25, Preston Hospital, Preston Road, North Shields.	North Shields 74101, ext. 258
South Shields	Clinic D, General Hospital.	South Shields 62649
Sunderland	Ward 17, General Hospital.	Sunderland 56256, ext. 338

Warwickshire

Leamington	Warneford General Hospital, Leamington Spa.	Leamington Spa 27121, ext. 292
Nuneaton	George Eliot Hospital, Nuneaton	Nuneaton 4201, ext. 268
Rugby	St. Cross Hospital, Barby Road, Rugby.	Rugby 72831

West Midlands

Birmingham	General Hospital, Birmingham.	(021) 236 8611, ext. 230/1 and 249
Coventry	Coventry and Warwickshire Hospital., Coventry.	(0203) 24055, ext. 242 and 243
Dudley	Guest Hospital, Dudley.	(0384) 53037
Walsall	Manor Hospital, Walsall.	Walsall 28911
Wolverhampton	The Royal Hospital, Wolverhampton.	Wolverhampton 51532, ext. 348/318

Wiltshire

Salisbury	General Infirmary, Salisbury.	Salisbury 5212, ext. 537
Swindon	Princess Margaret Hospital, Swindon.	Swindon 22568

Yorkshire–North

Harrogate	Harrogate District Hospital.	Harrogate 885959, ext. 56
Scarborough	St. Mary's Hospital, Scarborough.	Scarborough 76111, ext. 63
York	York District Hospital, York.	York 31313

Yorkshire–South

Barnsley	District Hospital, Barnsley.	Barnsley 82250
Doncaster	Royal Infirmary, Doncaster.	Doncaster 66666, ext. 14

List of clinics

Rotherham	Moorgate General Hospital, Rotherham.	Rotherham 2171, ext. 317
Sheffield	Royal Infirmary, Sheffield.	Sheffield 78981

Yorkshire-West

Bradford	St. Luke's Hospital, Bradford.	Bradford 34744, ext. 314/315
Dewsbury	General Hospital, Dewsbury.	Dewsbury 46511, ext. 21/27
Halifax	Royal Infirmary, Halifax.	Halifax 60234, ext. 238
Huddersfield	Royal Infirmary, Lindley, Huddersfield.	Huddersfield (0484) 22191, ext. 357/359
Keighley	Airedale General Hospital, Eastburn, Keighley.	Steeton 52511, ext. 284/5/6/7
Leeds	General Infirmary, Leeds.	0532 32799, ext. 279
Wakefield	Clayton Hospital, Wakefield.	Wakefield 75122, ext. 15/211

London Boroughs

Brent	Central Middlesex Hospital, NW10.	01–965 5733, ext. 632/633
Camden	University College Hospital, WC1.	01–387 9300, ext. 528/527
Camden	Royal Free Hospital. NW3 2QG	01–794 0500, ext. 3620/3619
City of London	St. Bartholomew's Hospital, EC1.	01–600 9000, ext. 555
City of London	St. Paul's Hospital, WC2.	01–836 9611
Croydon	General Hospital, Croydon, Surrey.	01–688 7755, ext. 333
Greenwich	Seamen's Hospital. SE10 9LE	01–858 3433, ext. 32
Hackney	Eastern Hospital. E9 6BY	01–985 1193, ext. 26/28
Hammersmith	West London Hospital, W6 7DQ	01–748 3441, ext. 10 and 102
Haringay	Prince of Wales General Hospital, Tottenham. N15 4AN	01–808 0550, 01–808 1081 ext. 229
Havering	Old Church Hospital, Romford.	Romford 46090, ext. 3258
Hillingdon	Hillingdon Hospital.	Uxbridge 38282, ext. 537 and 601
Hounslow	West Middlesex Hospital, Isleworth.	01–560 2121, ext. 425
Islington	Diagnostic Clinic, Moorfields Eye Hospital, City Road, EC1.	01-253 3411, or 222
Islington	Royal Northern Hospital. N7 6LD	01–272 7777, ext. 375
Kensington and Chelsea	St. Stephen's Hospital. SW10 9TH	01–352 8161, ext. 426 and 433
Kensington and Chelsea	St. Mary Abbots Hospital. W8 5LQ	01–937 8201, ext. 203

Lambeth	Lydia Department, St. Thomas's Hospital. SE1 7EH	01–928 9292, ext. 2129 and 2329
Lambeth	Alexandra Clinic, St. Giles' Hospital. SE5 7RN	01–703 0898, ext. 6024 and 6202
Lambeth	South London Hospital. SW4 9 DR	01–673 7788, ext. 319
Lewisham	St. John's Hospital. SE13 7NW	01–852 4467, ext. 27
Newham	Queen Mary's Hospital. E15 4SD	01–534 2616, ext. 7
Southwark	Lloyd Clinic, Guy's Hospital. SE1 9RT	01–407 7600, ext. 2292
Sutton	St. Helier Hospital, Carshalton.	01–644 4343, ext. 213
Tower Hamlets	Whitechapel Clinic, The London Hospital.	01–247 7310; 01–247 6436
Westminster	James Pringle House, Middlesex Hospital. W1N 8AA	01–636 8333, ext. 666 01–323 4819
Westminster	St. George's Hospital, Hyde Park Corner. SW1X 7EZ	01–235 4343, ext. 104
Westminster	Praed Street Clinic, St. Mary's Hospital. W2	01–262 1123
Westminster	Westminster Hospital, St. John's Gardens. SW1	01–828 9811, ext. 2225 and 2302

Northern Ireland

Health/social services area	*Address and telephone number of clinic*	
Eastern	Royal Victoria Hospital, Belfast.	Belfast 20159
Eastern	Ulster Hospital, Dundonald, Belfast.	Dundonald 2611
Eastern	Mater Infirmorum Hospital, Crumlin Road, Belfast.	Belfast 744474
Northern	Waveney Hospital, Ballymena.	Ballymena 6561
Northern	Coleraine Hospital, Coleraine.	Coleraine 3244
Southern	Daisy Hill Hospital, Newry.	Newry 3292
Western	Altnagelvin Hospital, Londonderry.	Londonderry 65171
Western	Erne Hospital, Enniskillen.	Enniskillen 4711
Western	Tyrone County Hospital, Omagh.	Omagh 2565

Scotland

County and town	*Address and telephone number of clinic*	
	Aberdeenshire	
Aberdeen	Royal Infirmary, Aberdeen.	Aberdeen 51104/23423, ext. 405

List of clinics

Angus

Dundee   55 Constitution Road, Dundee.   Dundee 23491, ext. 41 and 32

Ayrshire

Ayr   Heathfield Hospital, Ayr.   0292 68621

Dumfriesshire

Dumfries   Dumfries and Galloway Royal Infirmary, Dumfries.   Dumfries 3151 ext. 404

Fife

Dunfermline   Dunfermline and West Fife Hospital, Reid Street, Dunfermline.   Dunfermline 23131, ext. 31

Kirkcaldy   Victoria Hospital, Kirkcaldy.   Kirkcaldy 61155, ext. 42

Inverness-shire

Inverness   Raigmore Hospital, Inverness.   Inverness 34151, ext. 201/2

Inverness   Belford Hospital, Fort William.   Fort William 2481, ext. 41

Lanark

Glasgow   67 Black Street, Glasgow. G4 OEF   (041) 552 1529 (male)

Glasgow   Southern General Hospital, Glasgow. G51 4TF   (041) 445 2466

Glasgow   63 Black Street, Glasgow. G4 OEF   (041) 552 0680 (female)

Glasgow   Western Infirmary, Glasgow. G11 6NT   (041) 339 8822, ext. 529

Hamilton   Oak Lodge Special Clinic, Almada Lane, off Almada Street, Hamilton.   Hamilton 23459

Midlothian

Edinburgh   Royal Infirmary, Edinburgh.   Edinburgh (031) 229 2477, ext. 2144/2100

Perthshire

Perth   Royal Infirmary, Perth.   Perth 23311

Renfrew

Greenock   Royal Infirmary, Greenock.   (0475) 20374
Greenock   Gateside Hospital, Greenock.   (0475) 25252

Stirlingshire

Falkirk   Royal Infirmary, Falkirk.   Falkirk 23011, ext. 51
Stirling   Royal Infirmary, Stirling.   Stirling 3041, ext. 214

List of clinics
Wales

List of clinics

St. Helier
(Jersey)   General Hospital, St. Helier.   Central 24242, ext. 233

Isle of Man

County and town   *Address and telophone number of clinic*

Douglas   Noble's Isle of Man Hospital, Westmoreland Road, Douglas, Isle of Man.   Douglas (0624) 3661, ext. 25

Eire

County and town   *Address and telephone number of clinic*

Cork

County and town	Address	Telephone
Cork	City Hall, Cork.	Cork (021) 2278, ext. 20 (021) 21731 (021) 51588
Cork	St. Finbarr's Hospital, Cork.	Cork (021) 26721 (021) 35311

Dublin

County and town	Address	Telephone
Dublin	Mater Misericordiae Hospital, North Circular Road, Dublin.	Dublin 304488 and 301122
Dublin	Sir Patrick Dun's Hospital, Grand Canal Street, Dublin.	Dublin 766942, ext. 7
Dublin	Dr. Steeven's Hospital, Dublin.	Dublin 772606

Clare

Ennis	County Hospital, Ennis.	Ennis (065) 8713

Westmeath

Mullingar	County Hospital, Mullingar.	Mullingar (044) 80221

Waterford

Waterford	Ardkeen Hospital, Waterford.	Waterford (051) 3321

Index

G signifies entry in glossary

Index